Peterson's

MASTER THE

PANRE

2013

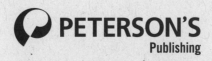

PETERSON'S
Publishing

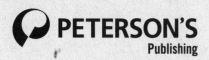

About Peterson's Publishing

To succeed on your lifelong educational journey, you will need accurate, dependable, and practical tools and resources. That is why Peterson's is everywhere education happens. Because whenever and however you need education content delivered, you can rely on Peterson's to provide the information, know-how, and guidance to help you reach your goals. Tools to match the right students with the right school. It's here. Personalized resources and expert guidance. It's here. Comprehensive and dependable education content— delivered whenever and however you need it. It's all here.

For more information, contact Peterson's, 2000 Lenox Drive, cqx, Lawrenceville, NJ 08648; 800-338-3282 Ext. 54229; or find us online at www.petersonspublishing.com.

Facebook® and Facebook logos are registered trademarks of Facebook, Inc. Facebook, Inc. was not involved in the production of this book and makes no endorsement of this product.

Bernadette Webster, Managing Editor; Ray Golaszewski, Publishing Operations Manager; Linda M. Williams, Composition Manager

ISBN-13: 978-0-7689-3616-2
ISBN-10: 0-7689-3616-0
Printed in the United States of America

10 9 8 7 6 5 4 3 2 1   14 13 12

First Edition

By printing this book on recycled paper (40% post-consumer waste) 28 trees were saved.

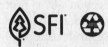

Contents

facebook.com/petersonspublishing

Before You Begin

OVERVIEW

- **Working as a physician assistant**
- **Becoming a physician assistant**
- **How this book is organized**

Congratulations on your decision to maintain your certification as a physician assistant (PA). By purchasing and using this guide, you are taking a very important step to furthering your career accomplishments.

Master the Physician Assistant National Recertification Examination (PANRE) will help you to prepare for this important test so that you may attain your best possible score and continue to practice as a certified physician assistant.

WORKING AS A PHYSICIAN ASSISTANT

Physician assistants are medical professionals formally trained and certified to provide medical and surgical services under a supervising physician or surgeon. As members of an organization's healthcare team, physician assistants provide a broad range of healthcare services to patients as regulated by state law and the supervising physician. They conduct physical exams, take medical histories, diagnose and treat illnesses, counsel patients, order and interpret laboratory tests, assist with surgeries, provide therapy, and prescribe medications.

There are many career pathways available for physician assistants. Some PAs work in the field of primary care, including family medicine, pediatrics, and internal medicine. Others are employed in specialty areas such as emergency medicine, geriatrics, orthopedics, and general and thoracic surgery. Physician assistants working in surgical units care for preoperative and postoperative patients or help surgeons as first or second assistants. PAs may also work for health maintenance organizations, public and private colleges and universities, and various government agencies.

Physician assistants practice autonomous decision making delegated by a physician to provide high-quality, professional medical care. Depending upon the workplace, some physician assistants have managerial responsibilities such as overseeing the work of medical technicians and ordering medical equipment and supplies. In some rural or inner-city facilities, physicians may not be on site or may only be available a limited number of hours. In these types of workplaces, physician assistants serve as principle care providers and confer with the supervising physician as needed.

According to the U.S. Bureau of Labor Statistics, employment prospects for physician assistants look very strong over the next decade. The field has seen dramatic growth in the past few years, and by 2018, jobs for physician assistants are expected to increase by 39 percent. As the healthcare industry continues to expand and associated costs continue to rise, healthcare providers are hiring more physician assistants to perform routine medical duties once performed exclusively by physicians. According to the Association of American Medical Colleges, a shortage of nearly 150,000 physicians is expected in the United States over the next 15 years. As certified healthcare professionals, physician assistants are expected to help narrow this gap and provide needed medical services as part of an organization's professional healthcare team.

BECOMING A PHYSICIAN ASSISTANT

All states require prospective physician assistants to complete a formal education program at an accredited institution and pass a national exam—the Physician Assistant National Certifying Examination (PANCE) for initial certification, and the Physician Assistant National Recertification Examination (PANRE) for recertification or certification maintenance. Both exams are administered by the National Commission on Certification of Physician Assistants (NCCPA). Only graduates of accredited physician assistant education programs are eligible to take these exams.

Most PA education programs take at least two years to complete for full-time students and require a bachelor's degree for admission. Admission to these programs is highly competitive, and most programs have prerequisites such as chemistry, anatomy, biology, microbiology, and physiology. Programs are structured on the basis of medical school curriculum, combining both classroom and clinical instruction. PA education programs are challenging and require intensive study. On average, programs take about 27 months to complete.

In addition to a college degree, many applicants to PA programs have experience in the healthcare field as emergency medical technicians, registered nurses, or paramedics. Physician assistant programs are offered by many four-year colleges, schools of allied health, academic health centers, or medical schools. Some PA programs may also be found at community colleges and hospitals or through the military.

Students in physician assistant educational programs receive both classroom and laboratory instruction in human anatomy, physiology, biochemistry, pathology, physiology, physical diagnosis, clinical medicine, and medical ethics. PA programs provide students with supervised clinical training in family medicine, surgery, internal medicine, prenatal care and gynecology, pediatrics, emergency medicine, and geriatrics.

Physician assistants may choose to continue their education in a particular specialty after graduating from an accredited program and obtaining certification through the NCCPA. Postgraduate programs for physician assistants are offered in a variety of medical fields, including emergency medicine, surgery, pediatrics, internal medicine, rural primary care, neonatology, and occupational medicine.

Credentials and Licensure

All fifty states and the District of Columbia have laws governing the practice of physician assistants. To obtain a license and use the credential, Physician Assistant-Certified (PA-C), all physician assistants must graduate from an accredited PA education program and pass a series of exams administered by the National Commission on Certification of Physician Assistants (NCCPA). They must take the Physician Assistant National Certifying Examination (PANCE) for initial certification and the Physician Assistant National Recertifying Examination (PANRE) every six years thereafter to maintain certification. In addition to these requirements, physician assistants must earn and log 100 hours of continuing medical education (CME) every two years.

HOW THIS BOOK IS ORGANIZED

To help you prepare for the PANRE as productively and efficiently as possible, this book has been carefully researched, written, and organized. Each chapter reviews important material that is likely to appear on the PANRE. Completing the comprehensive practice test in this book will help you pass this exam.

To get the most out of this book, take the time to read each section carefully and thoroughly.

- Part I provides an overview of the PANRE and the recertification process. It also offers information on topics related to physician assistant education and career pathways, licensure, certification, and testing policies. Part I outlines the steps you need to take to maintain your certification as a physician assistant, including applying for and taking the PANRE and the certification maintenance cycle.
- Part II is an overview of the types of questions you will see on the PANRE. A chapter is devoted to each subject area on the test. Each chapter begins with a review of the question type, tips for answering those particular questions, and practice questions with answer explanations. Complete the questions and study the answer explanations. Even if you answered the questions correctly, you may discover a new tip in the explanation that will help you answer other questions on the test correctly.
- Part III offers a study guide for PANRE candidates. Included in the section are tips and suggestions for the best ways to prepare for the exam, as well as a list of organ systems for test-takers to study and review.
- When you feel that you are well prepared, move on to Part IV—the Practice Test. The questions on the practice test in this book are similar to the actual questions that you will see on the exam. If possible, try to work through the entire exam in one sitting. The actual test is administered in 4 blocks of 60 questions, with 60 minutes allowed for each block. Do not look at the correct answer until you have completed the exam. Remember,

these tests are for practice; take the time to learn from your mistakes in order to improve in these areas.

- The Appendices in Part V offer supplementary information to help you prepare for the PANRE, including disorders tested on the PANRE, expanded and detailed information pertaining to organ systems, charts of infectious disease organisms, common medical abbreviations, and prescription abbreviations.

Special Advertising Section

At end of the book, don't miss the special section of ads placed by Peterson's preferred clients. Their financial support helps make it possible for Peterson's Publishing to continue to provide you with the highest-quality test preparation, educational exploration, and career preparation resources you need to succeed on your educational journey.

Find Us on Facebook

Join the career conversation on Facebook® at www.facebook.com/petersonspublishing and receive additional test-prep tips and advice. Peterson's resources are available to help you do your best on the PANRE and other important exams in your future.

Peterson's Publications

Peterson's publishes a full line of books—career preparation, test preparation, education exploration, and financial aid. Peterson's publications can be found at high school guidance offices, college libraries and career centers, and local bookstores and libraries. Peterson's books are now also available as eBooks.

We welcome any comments or suggestions you may have about this publication. Your feedback will help us make educational dreams possible for you—and others like you.

PART I

THE PANRE AND RECERTIFICATION

CHAPTER 1

About the PANRE

OVERVIEW

- What is tested on the PANRE?
- How the exam is developed
- How to register for the PANRE

Every six years, all physician assistants must take and pass the Physician Assistant National Recertifying Examination (PANRE) to maintain their certification to practice medicine. This test is developed and administered by the National Commission on Certification of Physician Assistants (NCCPA) and provides a comprehensive assessment of a practicing physician assistant's accumulated skills and knowledge base in the profession.

Consisting of 240 multiple-choice questions, the PANRE is computer-based and offered at Pearson VUE testing centers. The exam takes 4 hours to complete and is administered in four blocks of 60 questions. Sixty minutes are allocated for each block, with an additional 45 minutes given for break time between test blocks. Before the exam begins, test-takers view a 15-minute online tutorial. The cost for the PANRE is $350.

Physician assistants who do not pass the PANRE must wait 90 days to retake the exam, and they may only take the exam twice in one year.

WHAT IS TESTED ON THE PANRE?

Content Blueprint

Questions on the NCCPA's recertification exam, the PANRE, cover two domains: organ systems and task areas. The first domain, organ systems, tests candidates' knowledge of human organ systems and the various diseases, disorders, and diagnoses associated with those systems. The second domain—task areas—measures knowledge and skills acquired by physician assistants in relation to those diseases, disorders, and diagnoses.

Like the Physician Assistant National Certifying Examination (PANCE), subject areas covered on the PANRE focus on clinical and surgical knowledge and practice. However, questions on the PANRE tend to be of a more general nature. Physician assistants seeking recertification are expected to have the accumulated knowledge and skills to apply basic scientific concepts to broader clinical issues. Furthermore, many test questions are interrelated. For example, questions may test both medical knowledge and legal or ethical concerns, and up to one fifth of PANRE questions may relate in some manner to surgery.

The following list shows the organ systems and task areas included on the PANRE, as well as the percentage of the test's content allocated to these concepts.

Organ Systems

Cardiovascular—16%

- Cardiomyopathy; conduction disorders; congenital heart disease; heart failure; hypertension; hypotension; coronary heart disease; vascular disease; valvular disease; other forms of heart disease

Dermatologic—5%

- Eczematous eruptions; papulosquamous diseases; desquamation; vesicular bullae; acneiform lesions; verrucous lesions; insects/parasites; neoplasms; hair and nails; viral diseases; bacterial infections; fungal infections; other

EENT (Eyes, Ears, Nose, and Throat)—9%

- Eye disorders; ear disorders; nose/sinus disorders; mouth/throat disorders; benign and malignant neoplasms

Endocrine—6%

- Diseases of the thyroid gland; diseases of the adrenal glands; diseases of the pituitary gland; diabetes mellitus; lipid disorders

Gastrointestinal/Nutritional—10%

- Esophagus; stomach; gallbladder; pancreas; small intestine/colon; rectum; hernia; infectious and noninfectious diarrhea; vitamin and nutritional deficiencies; metabolic disorders

Genitourinary—6%

- GU tract conditions; infectious/inflammatory conditions; neoplastic diseases; renal diseases; fluid and electrolyte disorders; acid/base disorders

Hematologic—3%

- Anemias; coagulation disorders; malignancies

Infectious Diseases—3%

- Fungal disease; bacterial disease; mycobacterial disease; parasitic disease; spirochetal disease; viral disease

Musculoskeletal—10%

- Disorders of the shoulder; disorders of the forearm/wrist/hand; disorders of the back/spine; disorders of the hip; disorders of the knee; disorders of the ankle/foot; infectious diseases; neoplastic disease; osteoarthritis; osteoporosis; compartment syndrome; rheumatologic conditions

Neurologic System—6%

- Diseases of peripheral nerves; headaches; infectious disorders; movement disorders; vascular disorders; other neurologic disorders

Psychiatry/Behavioral—6%

- Anxiety disorders; attention-deficit/hyperactivity disorder (ADHD); autistic disorder; eating disorders; mood disorders; personality disorders; psychoses; somatoform disorders; substance use disorders; other behavior/emotional disorders

Pulmonary—12%

- Infectious disorders; neoplastic disease; obstructive pulmonary disease; pleural disease; pulmonary circulation; restrictive pulmonary disease; other pulmonary disease

Reproductive—8%

- Uterus; ovary; cervix; vagina/vulva; menstrual disorders; menopause; breast; pelvic inflammatory disease; contraceptive methods; infertility; uncomplicated pregnancy; complicated pregnancy

Task Areas

Using Laboratory and Diagnostic Studies—14%

History Taking and Performing Physical Examinations—16%

Formulating Most Likely Diagnosis—18%

Health Maintenance—10%

Clinical Intervention—14%

Pharmaceutical Therapeutics—18%

Applying Basic Science Concepts—10%

PANRE Subject Areas

The PANRE covers a wide range of subject areas to ensure that recertification candidates possess the needed medical and surgical knowledge to successfully treat patients in a variety of medical practice areas. Subject areas that are tested on the PANRE include the following:

- Anatomy and Physiology
- Bleeding Disorders
- CDC Prevention Isolation Guidelines
- Dementia
- HIV and AIDS
- Immune System
- Liver Function
- Maslow's Hierarchy of Needs
- Multiple Sclerosis
- Obstetrics and Gynecology
- Pharmacology
- Surgical Terminology

HOW THE EXAM IS DEVELOPED

PANRE test questions are developed following a rigorous and comprehensive review process. Practicing physicians and physician assistants are chosen to serve on test development committees for the National Commission on Certification of Physician Assistants (NCCPA) on the basis of their geographic locations, practice experience and specialties, and writing abilities. Test committees produce new sets of test questions, and these questions are subsequently reviewed by medical editors and content specialists for possible addition to the exam.

Questions that are recommended for future inclusion on the PANRE, known as pre-test items, are placed on the PANRE along with regularly scored questions. Examinees' responses allow the NCCPA to collect statistics pertaining to each new question and determine which questions meet examination criteria.

Exam Options

Practice-Focused Component

As you prepare to take the PANRE for recertification as a physician assistant, you will need to decide between the primary care option and an area of specialization, also known as the practice-focused component. These areas of specialization comprise 40 percent of the PANRE's content. The remaining 60 percent of the exam's content will cover generalist questions that are answered by all PANRE test-takers. Although all the questions on the PANRE are of a generalist nature, candidates may customize their exam depending on their area of practice and expertise. They may choose to take the PANRE in one of three formats, including primary care, adult medicine, and surgery.

Primary Care

If you decide to take the PANRE's standard exam format based on primary care, 100 percent of the test questions will fall under the generalist category.

Adult Medicine

If you choose to specialize in adult medicine, 60 percent of the PANRE will contain generalist questions related to primary care, and 40 percent of the PANRE will focus on questions pertaining to adult medicine. Questions are written by specialists in adult medicine and cover subjects such as endocrinology, cardiology, psychiatry, pulmonary medicine, rheumatology, and neurology.

Surgery

If you opt for the surgery specialization, 60 percent of the exam will consist of generalist questions related to primary care, and 40 percent of the PANRE will focus on questions pertaining to surgery. Questions are written by specialists in surgery and cover subjects such as general surgery, vascular surgery, plastic surgery, cardiac surgery, neurosurgery, orthopedic surgery, urology/nephrology surgery, thoracic surgery, and ENT surgery.

Choosing the Best PANRE Exam Option

Choosing an area of specialization for the PANRE is not required. Remember, regardless of what option you choose, the PANRE is a generalist exam testing clinical and surgical knowledge. Both the traditional and specialized exams cover the same content blueprint. If you select the primary care option, you will be taking the same PANRE that has been offered in years past. If you choose an area of specialization, 60 percent of your exam will follow the same content blueprint as the traditional PANRE, and 40 percent of the exam will include generalist questions specific to either adult medicine or surgery. By selecting the practice-focused exam, your exam will have more generalist questions in one of the two specialized areas.

Each version of the PANRE exam is designed to meet the same standard of difficulty. The practice-focused exams are not any easier or more difficult than the primary care exam, and both types of exams lead to the same credential. Just like primary care exams, practice-focused exams are scored as one examination with a single score, so there is no advantage or disadvantage to choosing a particular exam option. Score reports do not show areas of specialization, and no special recognition is given for choosing the practice-focused exam. Choosing the primary care, adult medicine, or surgery focus allows candidates for recertification to correlate their test-preparation studies and knowledge base with their practical work experience.

Exam Blocks

The PANRE exam consists of four blocks of 60 test questions. You will have 60 minutes to complete each block and are free to answer the questions within each block in any order. You are also permitted to change and review your responses to each question during the time alloted for each test block. Once you decide to exit a test block, or after the time designated for that block has expired, you will no longer be able to answer or review test questions or change your responses.

Exam Length

You will be given 4 hours to take the PANRE. The exam is comprised of 240 multiple-choice questions that are divided into four blocks of 60 questions each. Test-takers have 60 minutes to complete each block. In addition to time allotted for the exam, you will be allowed 45 minutes of break time between exam blocks, which you may manage however you choose. Before you begin taking the PANRE, you will complete an exam tutorial that takes 15 minutes.

Specialty Certificates of Added Qualifications (CAQs)

Physician assistants now have the opportunity to add a specialization to their credentials through a new program offered by the NCCPA: the Certificate of Added Qualifications (CAQ). This program allows physician assistants to be recognized with additional credentials in their specialty area of expertise, including emergency medicine, cardiovascular and thoracic surgery, nephrology, psychiatry, and orthopedic surgery. The CAQ program is voluntary and allows physician assistants to add professional credentials to their generalist certifications through the NCCPA.

To be eligible for the Certificate of Added Qualifications Program, physician assistants must possess both of the following:

1. Current certification as a PA-C

2. A valid and unrestricted license from at least one jurisdiction in the United States or its territories to practice as a physician assistant or an unrestricted privilege granted by a government agency to practice as a physician assistant

If a PA meets these necessary prerequisites, he or she may continue the CAQ process by completing these additional four requirements:

1. Continuing medical education (CME) in a Category I specialty

2. One to two years of relevant healthcare experience

3. Appropriate patient case and procedures experience within the chosen specialty

4. Passing score on a specialty exam (taken after the other three requirements are met)

CAQ exams are 2 hours long and consist of 120 multiple-choice questions. The test is divided into two blocks of 60 questions, and 60 minutes are allotted to each test block.

HOW TO REGISTER FOR THE PANRE

Exam Eligibility

Applicants for recertification are evaluated by the National Commission on Certification of Physician Assistants (NCCPA) and are not discriminated against on the basis of gender, race, age, sexual orientation, national origin, religion, disability, or marital status. In order to take the PANRE, you must meet the eligibility requirements specified by the NCCPA. Certified physician assistants are eligible to take the PANRE if they meet one of the following requirements:

1. The physician assistant is in the fifth or sixth year of the certification maintenance cycle.

2. The physician assistant has fulfilled the requirements to regain certification by taking the PANRE.

The NCCPA strictly enforces and will not waive exam eligibility requirements. Scores for exams taken by ineligible applicants as determined by the NCCPA either will not be reported or will be rescinded.

At any one time, test-takers may only be registered for a single NCCPA exam. Exam applicants wishing to take the PANRE may only take this test once during a 90-day period, and they may only attempt the exam twice each calendar year—twice during the fifth year and twice in the sixth year of the certification maintenance cycle.

Once you have applied to take the PANRE, you will be given 180 days to take the exam from the start of your designated exam timeframe. You will receive an e-mail acknowledgment of your exam application from the NCCPA listing these dates. One exception to this policy is for individuals applying to take the PANRE late in the sixth year of their certification maintenance cycle. In this case, the exam timeframe will be fewer than 180 days and will end on the last exam administration date for the year that certification expires.

PANRE Registration

Once you have submitted your registration materials successfully, the NCCPA will send you an acknowledgment e-mail establishing your 180-day timeframe to take the exam. You may then check the availability of your preferred testing center and schedule the PANRE at a convenient time. The PANRE is administered at over 200 testing sites, so you should be able to choose one that is in proximity to where you live and work.

To register for the PANRE, you will need to submit the following materials to NCCPA:

- A completed online application
- A $350 application fee

Special Testing Accommodations

In compliance with the Americans with Disabilities Act (ADA) and the ADA Amendments Act of 2008 (ADAAA), the NCCPA makes reasonable efforts to accommodate test-takers with documented disabilities and other qualifying medical conditions. A disability is defined by the ADAAA as a physical or mental impairment that limits major life activities in a significant way as compared to an average individual without these restrictions. The NCCPA will provide special testing accommodations to these individuals while maintaining the security and integrity of the exam, including the use of medication, medical devices, or auxiliary aides and services. Decisions as to which ADA-covered medical conditions will be accommodated are at the NCCPA's discretion.

Test-takers with a documented disability recognized by the ADA should request special testing accommodations as early in the application process as possible by completing the request form included in the application materials. Additionally, examinees requiring special testing accommodations will need to provide supporting documentation to the NCCPA along with their registration materials or very soon after applying to take the PANRE.

For detailed guidelines explaining special accommodations for the exam and the required documentation, please visit the NCCPA Web site. Any delays in sending this documentation to the NCCPA will result in delays in completing the application process and in scheduling the exam, so applicants requesting special accommodations for the PANRE should be sure to send their request forms and submit their supporting documentation to the NCCPA as soon as possible.

Financial Policies

Fees

When you submit your application form to register for the PANRE, you must also pay the exam fee, which is currently $350. Exam fees must be paid in U.S. dollars and should accompany your application for the PANRE. Applications for the exam are not processed until payment has been received. In addition, all fees owed to the NCCPA, including current or past-due charges, must be paid before an application for the PANRE will receive final approval.

Declined credit cards, credit card charge backs, and returned checks will result in a $35 service charge by the NCCPA. In addition, the NCCPA will charge a $50 fee to issue replacement certificates to replace lost certificates or to reflect name changes or changes of address. Exam scores will only be released after all fees have been paid, including recent charges you may have incurred after your exam application was processed.

Applicants who fail to take the PANRE on their designated exam date or do not finish each of the required sections of the test will not have their exam fee refunded. Instead, those applicants will be required to reapply for the PANRE and will have to pay the exam fee at the time of their new application.

Withdrawals and Cancellations

If you are unable to take the PANRE on your scheduled test date that falls within the 180-day timeframe specified on the exam acknowledgement e-mail, you will need to contact the NCCPA in writing, either by mail, fax, or e-mail. In your written communication, you must request the withdrawal of your application and eligibility for the PANRE from your scheduled exam timeframe. This correspondence must be received by the NCCPA before the end date specified on your exam acknowledgement e-mail and at least one business day before your scheduled exam time with the testing center.

If you need to cancel or reschedule your exam, be sure to follow these guidelines. Otherwise, you will forfeit the $350 exam fee and will have to reapply for the PANRE. Remember, canceling your exam with the testing center is not the same procedure as withdrawing from your exam timeframe. To withdraw from your exam timeframe (and avoid having to reapply for the PANRE and forfeit your exam fee), you must contact the NCCPA directly.

Refunds

If you decide to withdraw from your PANRE exam timeframe and follow the procedures outlined above, your examination fee will be refunded. The NCCPA will send a refund directly to the person who made the exam fee payment.

Physician Assistant Recertification

OVERVIEW

- **Certification exams**
- **When to take the test**
- **Testing policies and procedures**
- **Test day procedures**

CERTIFICATION EXAMS

Graduates from physician assistant programs accredited by the Accreditation Review Commission on Education for the Physician Assistant (ARC-PA) must take and pass a series of examinations administered by the National Commission on Certification of Physician Assistants (NCCPA) to become certified physician assistants. The two examinations required by the NCCPA for certification are the Physician Assistant National Certifying Examination (PANCE) and the Physician Assistant National Recertifying Examination (PANRE).

The PANCE assesses medical and surgical knowledge in a multiple-choice format. Physician assistants who pass this exam receive initial NCCPA certification as well as the Physician Assistant-Certified (PA-C) credential. During their fifth or sixth year of practice, physician assistants must take the NCCPA exam for recertification, the PANRE. Like the PANCE, the PANRE tests clinical and surgical knowledge in a multiple-choice format. However, PAs taking the PANRE may choose from several different exam options, including the primary care option and one of two practice-focused exams in either adult medicine or surgery.

Maintaining Certification

In order to maintain their certification, physician assistants follow a six-year certification maintenance cycle consisting of three two-year periods. After passing the PANCE, certified physician assistants must earn at least 100 hours of continuing medical education (CME) and log these hours for each of the two-year periods. More information about CME is detailed in the section below titled, "CME Guidelines and Certification." Physician assistants may start accumulating CME hours on May 1 of the first year of the certification cycle and must complete these hours by December 31 of the second certification cycle year.

The certification maintenance cycle is strictly enforced with the only exception given to physician assistants who are earning and logging CME hours for the first time following certification. In this case, if the certification is issued after June 30, first-time loggers may request an extension for obtaining their CME requirement. Before the end of each two-year period, referred to as the certification expiration year, PA-Cs must send a certification maintenance fee, currently $130, to the NCCPA.

By the end of the six-year cycle, physician assistants must take and pass the PANRE for recertification. Once all the requirements for CME have been met and both exams have been passed, physician assistants begin the certification maintenance cycle again. To maintain certification as a PA-C, physician assistants must take and pass the PANRE every six years throughout the course of their professional careers.

Lost Certification

If certification is not maintained, physician assistants may choose from the following options to regain their lost credential:

- Physician assistants may take and pass the PANCE by applying for the exam online and submitting the test payment. For this option, CME hours are not required.

- Physician assistants may take and pass the PANRE. For this option, CME hours are required.

To regain certification by taking and passing the PANRE, physician assistants must submit an online application and payment for the exam. In addition, candidates for recertification must have logged 300 hours of CME within the last six years, with 100 of these hours earned during the last two years from the date of their exam application.

There are very specific requirements for logging CME hours for physician assistants who are trying to regain lost certification. Hours must be submitted to NCCPA using the CME Logging for Regaining Form, which may be found in the *CME Regaining Package* available on the NCCPA's Web site. Furthermore, at least half of the required CME hours (150 hours or more) must fall under Category I, and 50 of these Category I hours must have been earned within the two years prior to a candidate's online application and payment for the PANRE. CME hours will be reviewed and processed by the NCCPA after an applicant for recertification has applied to take the PANRE for recertification.

CME Guidelines and Certification

Continuing medical education (CME) hours are an essential part of earning and maintaining certification through the NCCPA. CME allows physician assistants to develop and enhance their knowledge and skills in order to provide the best service to patients. All certified physician assistants are required to earn and log 100 CME hours in the second, fourth, and sixth year of their certification maintenance cycle through continued clinical and professional education. These hours must be sent to the NCCPA online and be accompanied by a $130 certification maintenance fee.

CME hours are grouped under several different categories, including Certification Program, Category I, and Category II. For the certification process, physician assistants must earn and log at least 50 Category I continuing medical education hours as part of the 100-hour requirement every two years. Category I, or preapproved CME, includes credit programs that have been approved by the American Academy of Physician Assistants (AAPA), the American Academy of Family Physicians (AAFP), the American Osteopathic Association (AOA), and the American Medical Association (AMA). Category II, or elective CME, includes practice-related activities that are not eligible for Category I credit, such as postgraduate courses, independent study, and other programs.

The timeframe for completing and logging CME hours begins on May 1 of the year that certification was issued and ends on December 31 of the certification expiration year. For instance, if your certification expires in 2015, you will need to earn and log your CME between May 1, 2013 and December 31, 2015. For those who have just passed the PANCE, however, earning and logging CME hours may begin on the date that certification was issued.

CME Audits

To maintain the integrity of the continuing medical education (CME) requirement for all certified physician assistants, the NCCPA follows a regular schedule of audits for Category I hours. After completing their two-year certification maintenance cycle, randomly selected physician assistants are chosen to undergo an audit of their CME hours.

Those who are chosen for a random audit are required to send the necessary documentation supporting their earned and logged Category I hours to the NCCPA for review. If a physician assistant's CME hours cannot be verified or were falsely approved or reported as Category I credit, he or she will remain certified but must undergo another audit during the next two-year certification maintenance cycle. Furthermore, the physician assistant must meet two additional requirements before his or her current NCCPA certificate expires:

1. Replace any unsubstantiated Category I CME hours with documented and approved Category I CME hours

2. Pay a $100 re-audit fee to the NCCPA

If all of the above requirements are not met before the conclusion of the certificate expiration year, the physician assistant will lose his or her certification. Physician assistants who meet these requirements and maintain their certification during their second audit will face an additional random audit during one or more of their next three certification maintenance cycles to ensure their Category I CME hours are appropriately documented and valid.

CME audits are not optional. Physician assistants who do not respond to an audit notification letter within six weeks or refuse to have their Category I CME hours audited may have their certification immediately revoked by the NCCPA. Falsified documents or any other fraudulent reporting of Category I CME hours will also result in the loss of certification.

WHEN TO TAKE THE TEST

Scheduling the Exam

Physician assistants seeking recertification may take the PANRE twice in the fifth year and twice in the sixth year of their certification maintenance cycle. There is a mandatory waiting period of 90 days between exam attempts for candidates who do not pass the exam.

As soon as you become eligible to take the PANRE, you should schedule your test date with your preferred testing center in order to secure the location and date most convenient for you. After you successfully submit your application materials, the NCCPA will send you an acknowledgement e-mail indicating your 180-day exam timeframe and providing instructions for scheduling your exam date.

It is a good idea to arrive at the testing center early to avoid any last-minute delays or other stress-inducing situations. If you are late for the exam, you will not be permitted to take the PANRE and will have to reapply to take the test and forfeit your exam fee. Plan to be at the testing site 30 minutes before your scheduled exam time on the test date.

Once you have started to take the PANRE, you must stay for the duration of the exam and finish the entire test. The NCCPA does not refund the exam fee or give credit toward future exam fees should you fail to complete the PANRE.

Rescheduling or Canceling the Exam

Remember, if you are registered to take the PANRE but do not take the test during your designated exam timeframe, you will lose your exam fee and must reapply to take the PANRE. If you decide to reschedule or cancel your exam, you must contact the NCCPA in writing via e-mail, fax, or mail to request the withdrawal of your PANRE application and eligibility from your designated 180-day timeframe. You will also need to contact the testing center 24 hours before your scheduled exam date to inform them of the cancellation. These procedures must be followed to avoid losing your exam fee and having to reapply to take the PANRE.

Exam Deadlines

To take the PANRE on your preferred date, you will need to submit all of your application materials (including the online application and the exam fee) to the NCCPA before the published deadline. Exam deadlines are updated regularly and may be found on the NCCPA's Web site. Once the NCCPA receives your materials, a notice of your eligibility will be sent to Pearson VUE, and your exam date will be scheduled.

How Often May the Test Be Taken?

Physician assistants seeking recertification through the PANRE must adhere to several requirements when scheduling the exam, including the following:

- Test-takers may attempt the PANRE only once during any 90-day period.
- The PANRE may be taken twice during the fifth year and twice during the sixth year of a candidate's certification maintenance cycle.
- Examinees are given an exam timeframe of up to 180 days as specified in their exam acknowledgement e-mail from the NCCPA.

TESTING POLICIES AND PROCEDURES

Identification Requirements

To be admitted to the test center, you will be asked to show two forms of identification that are both valid and current. Your two forms of identification must include the following:

1. Photo identification with both your signature and printed name

2. Another form of identification with your signature and printed name

Be sure to let the NCCPA know right away if you have a name change prior to the exam so that your record is updated before your test date. The names on your two forms of identification must match the name that the NCCPA has for you on record. If the names do not match or if you do not bring the two required forms of identification, you will not be allowed to take the exam. In this case, you will forfeit your exam fee and will have to reapply to take the PANRE.

Personal Belongings

When you arrive at the testing center, you will need to secure all personal belongings in an assigned locker and will not be permitted to bring any items into the testing room. Personal belongings include purses, tote bags, cell phones, computers, books, notes, hats, watches, pagers, cameras, recorders, food, and beverages. You will be able to retrieve these items during scheduled break times, but they must be returned to your locker before you resume taking the PANRE. Do not bring NCCPA examination materials with you to the testing center because they will be confiscated. Your personal belongings and their contents may be inspected if there is reason for suspicion.

If you require the use of medical equipment or devices during the exam, you will need to make arrangements to do so in advance with the NCCPA by requesting special testing accommodations. Please see the information in Chapter 1 under the heading "Special Testing Accommodations" for more information.

Written Notes

Examinees are not allowed to record or make written notes of the PANRE's contents. Taking notes during the exam is only permitted in the testing room using the center's laminated noteboards, which are permanent fixtures in the testing room and are erasable.

Examination Grievances and Appeals

In the unlikely event that you encounter unusual testing conditions or events that you believe had a negative effect on your exam performance, you may follow an established procedure with the NCCPA to file a grievance. A grievance must be submitted to the NCCPA within three business days of your exam and should include a signed and dated letter describing the adverse testing conditions. Any supporting documentation related to the incident should also be submitted. If your exam grievance is approved, your scores will be invalidated and you will need to reschedule the PANRE to meet this requirement for recertification.

If you are not successful in filing a grievance, you may follow an appeal process to have the decision reviewed by the NCCPA. To initiate a review of the decision or a policy exception, you will need to send the NCCPA a signed, written request, along with any related documentation supporting your appeal. The NCCPA will review your request and provide written notice of the outcome. If the NCCPA's decision is not in your favor, you will also receive a copy of the *Appeal Process for Adverse Certification Decisions,* which explains how further reviews of the decision are conducted. If you plan to file an additional Request for Review, this must be done within 30 days after receiving the written notice of the review outcome.

TEST DAY PROCEDURES

Arrival

Examinees should take care to arrive at the testing center early on their exam date. You should plan to be at the testing center at least 30 minutes before your scheduled exam time to avoid any last-minute complications or delays. If you are late for the exam, you may be refused admittance to the testing center and will not be allowed to take the PANRE, resulting in a forfeited exam fee and the necessity of reapplying for the exam. You will be expected to show two valid and current forms of identification, and your photograph will be taken at the testing center along with a digital fingerprint or palm scan.

Instruction

After you are admitted to the testing center and your identification is verified, testing center staff will explain how the computer equipment is used to administer the PANRE. Before your test session begins, you will complete a 15-minute tutorial to ensure that you understand how to take the exam. Test center staff remain at the center for the duration of the exam. With the help of recording equipment as well as video and audio monitors, test center staff are responsible for managing the exam process and observing test-takers to make sure that all exams are conducted fairly and consistently.

Breaks

The PANRE consists of four 60-minute blocks, and test-takers are permitted to take 45 minutes of scheduled break time between exam blocks. After each exam block is completed, examinees are notified of the opportunity for scheduled break time by a notice on their computer screens containing break instructions. Even if you do not feel tired or in need of a break, it is usually a good idea to take advantage of the scheduled break time offered between exam blocks to give your mind a short rest, stretch your legs, and relax for a few minutes before starting the next section of the exam. However, be sure to carefully follow the break instructions and keep your scheduled break time to 45 minutes or less over the course of the exam. If you take more than 45 minutes for scheduled breaks, these extra minutes will be deleted from your available exam time, and you will have less time to answer test questions.

It is also possible to take unscheduled breaks during exam blocks, but this is discouraged. Unscheduled break time will be subtracted from the work time you have available on that particular exam block, so you will have fewer minutes to complete that set of test questions. Ultimately, you are responsible for how you manage your break time, so try to use it wisely using the on-screen clocks provided. Think about how you can best arrange your break time in order to stay alert and focused for the entire exam. Spacing your breaks evenly is usually a good strategy since taking longer breaks early in the exam will leave you with little or no breaks between later exam blocks.

When you take a scheduled exam break, you will be allowed to leave and reenter the testing room, and you will have access to personal items stored in your assigned locker. Personal items may not be used during unscheduled breaks unless you have made arrangements for special testing conditions with the NCCPA in advance. Security is strictly maintained for scheduled break time, and you will be required to have a digital fingerprint or palm scan each time you leave and reenter the exam room.

Irregular Behavior

All NCCPA exams are closely monitored to ensure high testing standards. Testing center staff provide instructions to test-takers and carefully manage and observe test conditions. If the staff notice that an examinee does not follow instructions or proper test procedures, they may consider this to be irregular behavior. Test center staff are not required to inform test-takers if they observe irregular behavior, but the behavior will be reported to the NCCPA.

The NCCPA defines irregular behavior as any behavior that in some way invalidates or harms the integrity of the application, testing, or certification processes. These behaviors may occur during an exam, or they might take place before or after an exam. Irregular behavior includes, but is not limited to, the following actions:

- Possessing test materials prior to the exam

- Impersonating a test-taker

- Arranging for someone else take the exam for you

- Cheating on the exam by copying or exchanging answers

- Writing notes or possessing unauthorized materials (such as reference materials or recording devices) while taking a computer-based exam

- Reproducing test questions or stealing exam materials

- Altering NCCPA exam scores

- Falsifying NCCPA documents or certification

- Representing oneself as Physician Assistant-Certified (PA-C) without NCCPA certification

If the NCCPA determines that irregular behavior has taken place before, during, or after an examination, test-takers who engaged in dishonest or disruptive behavior may be disqualified from taking the PANRE or completing the exam. Their scores may be revoked, or they may be asked to retake the exam. Based on the nature of the offense, the NCCPA may take further disciplinary actions and impose sanctions against the offender. These sanctions may include legal action, fines, certificate suspension or revocation, and removal of eligibility for future exams or certificates. More detailed information regarding irregular behavior and the resulting disciplinary actions is described in the NCCPA publication, *Policies and Procedures for Disciplinary Review*.

Exam Scoring

About two weeks after taking the PANRE, the NCCPA will notify you by e-mail that it has received your exam results and will post your score to your personal certification record. However, if you owe the NCCPA any fees for current or past-due charges, you will not receive your exam score until these have been paid. You may also request a printed copy of your PANRE score by contacting the NCCPA.

The PANRE exam is scored using a systematic process that is designed to ensure accuracy and fairness. Test-takers are given one point for each correct answer and zero points for incorrect answers to produce a total score, called the raw score. Raw scores are calculated by two separate computer systems and then undergo an estimation procedure to produce an examinee's proficiency measure. This procedure helps to eliminate any disparity between different versions of the PANRE and compensate for any minor differences in the level of difficulty. Proficiency measures are then converted to scaled scores ranging from 200 to 800.

Unlike in years past, the NCCPA does not publish what percentage of questions must be answered correctly to pass the exam. Since there are multiple versions of the PANRE, the percentage may vary from one test to another. Instead, the NCCPA bases its passing or failing determinations on scaled scores and sets the passing standard based on that scale.

Scores may also be reported as invalid, meaning they are neither passing nor failing scores. Invalid scores may occur if a statistical analysis of a group of examinees reveals irregularities, such as inconsistencies in the exam administration or irregular behavior suspected of one or more test-takers. In these cases, scores may be held, rescinded, or determined to be invalid, depending on the outcome of a thorough review of the situation by the NCCPA.

PART II

OVERVIEW OF QUESTION TYPES

CHAPTER 3

Using Laboratory and Diagnostic Studies Questions

OVERVIEW

- **Preparing for using laboratory and diagnostic studies questions**
- **Tips for answering using laboratory and diagnostic studies questions**
- **Practice questions**
- **Answer key and explanations**
- **Summing it up**

PREPARING FOR USING LABORATORY AND DIAGNOSTIC STUDIES QUESTIONS

The first questions you will find on the PANRE are those that refer to laboratory and diagnostic studies. These questions are designed to test your knowledge of the various laboratory and diagnostic procedures used in the medical field and your ability to use them properly. This group of questions makes up 14 percent of the exam or about 34 items.

The using laboratory and diagnostic studies domain of the PANRE may include questions based on a variety of topics, such as:

- types of laboratory and diagnostic procedures;
- indications and contraindications for procedures;
- relevant procedures for selected conditions;
- safe and appropriate use of diagnostic equipment;
- collection, interpretation, and use of normal and abnormal diagnostic data;
- risks associated with laboratory and diagnostic procedures;
- cost effectiveness of selected procedures; and
- patient education regarding laboratory and diagnostic procedures.

Diagnosis is a critical element in the treatment of disease and injury. Developing an accurate, detailed picture of the patient's condition is crucial for developing and implementing the safest and most effective treatment possible. Often, visual observation and verbal communication alone are not enough to establish a definitive diagnosis. In such cases, physician assistants need to rely upon laboratory work and other forms of diagnostic testing in order to fully analyze the patient's condition and articulate a proper diagnosis. As a result, it is very important for physician assistants to have a strong understanding of the types of laboratory and other diagnostic tests used on a regular basis.

When preparing for the *using laboratory and diagnostic studies questions* you will encounter on the PANRE, you should be familiar with all of the different laboratory tests and diagnostic procedures you will have at your disposal as a physician assistant. Be sure that you understand what information these tests and procedures are designed to provide, which types of diagnostic procedures are most appropriate for use with a given condition, and how to use diagnostic equipment properly. You should also be familiar with the potential risks associated with these procedures and know when you should or should not use a particular procedure.

The PANRE may also contain questions that pertain to your ability to effectively communicate with your patients about the laboratory tests and diagnostic studies they are to undergo. Such questions will likely involve discussing specific instructions for a given procedure, explaining how a procedure works, obtaining the patient's consent, and more.

The multiple-choice questions on the PANRE will require you to choose the correct answer from a field of five choices.

TIPS FOR ANSWERING USING LABORATORY AND DIAGNOSTIC STUDIES QUESTIONS

When you are taking the PANRE, you may find it helpful to remember these hints:

1. Remember the purposes of common laboratory and diagnostic procedures. The most important parts of these questions are the laboratory and diagnostic procedures themselves. Understanding what these procedures are designed to do and how they work is critically important. When you are asked to choose the most appropriate procedure to use in a given situation, quickly scan the answer choices and eliminate any procedures that would not help you arrive at a diagnosis.

2. The patient's condition should dictate which procedure you use. Though there are many different types of laboratory and diagnostic procedures that can help you to formulate an accurate diagnosis, the choice of which procedure to use is not meant to be made randomly. When you are faced with a question that asks you to choose the most appropriate procedure for a particular patient, be sure to read carefully and pay close attention to all of the information it gives you about the patient's condition. This information should guide you toward the correct answer.

3. Remember when you should or should not use a certain procedure. Again, as you read the question, pay close attention to details about the patient's condition. In most cases, the patient's signs and symptoms will be an important factor in choosing the most appropriate procedure. Look for any signs or symptoms that indicate or contraindicate a certain procedure and make sure that you choose the safest and most effective procedure for the patient at hand.

Common laboratory and diagnostic studies are:

- Blood tests
- Auscultation
- X-rays
- CT scan
- Echocardiography
- Electrocardiography
- MRI
- Ultrasound
- Urinalysis

PRACTICE QUESTIONS

Directions: Choose the option that best answers the question.

1. A 13-year-old male presents with complaints of dizziness, shortness of breath, headaches, nose-bleeds, and chest pain. You suspect this is due to the congenital heart defect coarctation of the aorta. Which of the following imaging modalities would you suggest to confirm this diagnosis?
   (A) Echocardiogram
   (B) Myocardial perfusion imaging
   (C) Chest X-ray
   (D) Magnetic resonance angiography
   (E) MUGA scan

2. A 45-year-old African-American male with a history of uncontrolled hypertension presents with sudden, intense, stabbing pain in the back. Blood pressure is 220/110 mmHg, electrocardiogram is normal, troponin levels are normal, and d-dimer is normal. Which diagnostic procedure would you perform immediately?
   (A) CT scan of the chest to rule out pulmonary embolism
   (B) Lung V/Q scan to rule out pulmonary embolism
   (C) Echocardiogram to rule out pericarditis
   (D) Myocardial perfusion imaging to rule out cardiac ischemia
   (E) CT scan to rule out aortic dissection

3. A potassium hydroxide (KOH) smear would be a useful tool to confirm the diagnosis of which of the following dermatologic conditions?
   (A) Onychomycosis
   (B) Alopecia
   (C) Rosacea
   (D) Dyshidrosis
   (E) Psoriasis

4. A hydrogen breath test is the easiest and most reliable method to diagnose which of the following disorders?
   (A) Lactose intolerance
   (B) Celiac disease
   (C) *H. Pylori* infection
   (D) Irritable bowel syndrome
   (E) Gastritis

5. In order to accurately diagnose the condition of pertussis, which of the following specimens must be analyzed by a laboratory?
   (A) Blood
   (B) Saliva
   (C) Stool
   (D) Urine
   (E) Mucous

ANSWER KEY AND EXPLANATIONS

| 1. D | 2. E | 3. A | 4. A | 5. E |

1. **The correct answer is (D).** Coarctation of the aorta can be accurately diagnosed with magnetic resonance angiography. Echocardiograms may not be conclusive for teenagers and adults. In adults with untreated coarctation, blood often reaches the lower body through collaterals, e.g., internal thoracic arteries via the subclavian arteries. Those can be seen on MR or CT angiography.

2. **The correct answer is (E).** Aortic dissection is a tear or partial tear in the aorta, which is the largest blood vessel in the body. This condition is most common in individuals with uncontrolled hypertension and presents as a sudden, intense, stabbing pain in the back. This is an extremely emergent condition; therefore, if aortic dissection is suspected, a CT scan is recommended immediately in order to confirm or nullify the diagnosis.

3. **The correct answer is (A).** Onychomycosis is a fungal infection of the nails of the fingers or toes. A KOH preparation would be a useful tool to confirm the diagnosis of this disorder because it is used to confirm the presence of fungi.

4. **The correct answer is (A).** The hydrogen breath test is the most convenient and reliable test for lactase deficiency and lactose intolerance. For the breath test, pure lactose, usually 25 grams (the equivalent of 16 oz. of milk) is ingested with water after an overnight fast. In persons who are lactose intolerant, the lactose that is not digested and absorbed in the small intestine reaches the colon where the bacteria split the lactose into glucose and galactose and produce hydrogen (and/or methane) gas.

5. **The correct answer is (E).** In order for pertussis to be accurately diagnosed, a sample of mucous obtained from nasal passages must be collected and sent to a laboratory for analysis.

SUMMING IT UP

- Using laboratory and diagnostic studies questions will require an understanding of laboratory and diagnostic procedures; the indications and contraindications for these procedures; relevant procedures for selected conditions; safe and appropriate use of diagnostic equipment; the collection, interpretation, and use of normal and abnormal diagnostic data; the risks associated with specific procedures; the cost effectiveness of diagnostic procedures; and patient education regarding laboratory and diagnostic procedures.

- When studying for these questions, pay close attention to what each procedure is used for, how it works, what kind of data it should yield, the potential risks associated with it, and more. You will need to have a very strong understanding of the various diagnostic procedures you would be likely to use as a physician assistant.

- Pay close attention to the details. Many of these questions will provide you with specific information about the patient's condition. Be sure to read this information carefully and pay attention to the specific details related to the patient's presentation. You will need to know as much about the patient's condition as possible before you choose a course of action, so make sure to carefully take all of the patient's signs and symptoms into consideration.

- When you prepare for questions related to patient education regarding laboratory and diagnostic procedures, make sure that you understand the procedures involved well enough to be able to properly inform your patient about the procedure you want to perform, how it works, what it is designed to do, the possible risks, the potential benefits, and so on. Be sure that you are able to explain this information in a clear and concise manner that the patient can easily understand.

CHAPTER 4

History Taking and Performing Physical Examinations Questions

OVERVIEW

- **Preparing for history taking and performing physical examinations questions**
- **Tips for answering history taking and performing physical examinations questions**
- **Practice questions**
- **Answer key and explanations**
- **Summing it up**

PREPARING FOR HISTORY TAKING AND PERFORMING PHYSICAL EXAMINATIONS QUESTIONS

History taking and performing physical examinations questions are a second type of question on the PANRE. The questions pertaining to history taking and performing physical examinations will test your knowledge of a variety of issues related to interviewing and examining patients and reviewing their medical histories. This group of questions makes up 16 percent of the exam or about 38 items.

The history taking and performing physical examinations domain of the PANRE may include questions based on a variety of topics, such as:

- conducting thorough interviews;
- recognizing relevant historical data;
- performing thorough physical examinations;
- relating presenting complaints with medical history;
- recognizing relevant physical examination findings;
- associating historical data with selected conditions;
- recognizing risk factors for selected conditions;
- recognizing common signs and symptoms of selected conditions;
- techniques for performing physical examinations;

- conducting an appropriate physical exam directed toward a specific condition; and

- making a differential diagnosis based on presenting symptoms or exam findings.

Taking patient histories and performing physical examinations are among the most important parts of providing quality medical care. The information you gather from medical histories and physical examinations plays a crucial role in formulating an accurate diagnosis and choosing the most appropriate course of treatment. With this in mind, it is very important for physician assistants to be adequately skilled in this domain.

History taking and performing physical examinations questions are designed to test your understanding of concepts like conducting interviews, identifying relevant historical and physical examination data, performing comprehensive physical examinations, and correlating patient complaints with historical information. Some of the specific topics that are covered in this domain include historical information related to specific medical conditions, risk factors for specific conditions, typical signs and symptoms of specific conditions, examination techniques, typical examination findings related to specific conditions, appropriate physical examinations directed to specific conditions, and differential diagnoses related to presenting symptoms or physical observations.

When you prepare for the history taking and performing physical examinations domain, you should be sure that you have a firm understanding of the appropriate techniques for researching and utilizing patient medical histories and conducting thorough, focused physical examinations.

The multiple-choice questions on the PANRE will require you to choose the correct answer from a field of five choices.

TIPS FOR ANSWERING HISTORY TAKING AND PERFORMING PHYSICAL EXAMINATIONS QUESTIONS

When you are taking the PANRE, you may find it helpful to remember these hints:

1. Pay close attention to details. History taking and performing physical examinations questions will provide you with important details that you need to recognize and take into consideration before choosing the correct answer. Be sure to pay special attention to key details, such as signs, symptoms, complaints, findings, and so on.

2. Remember that your ultimate goal is diagnosis. Although the questions in this domain focus primarily on the methods and techniques for gathering information about your patients, it is important to remember that your goal in this process is to arrive at a diagnosis of the patient's condition. As you answer history taking and performing physical examinations questions, it may be helpful to keep this goal in mind.

PRACTICE QUESTIONS

Directions: Choose the option that best answers the question.

1. A 48-year-old female presents with dizziness, hearing loss, and drainage of the left ear. Examination of the ear revealed a type of skin cyst in the middle ear. Based on this examination, which of the following is the proper diagnosis?
   (A) Acoustic neuroma
   (B) Hemangioma
   (C) Hematoma
   (D) Cholesteatoma
   (E) Tympanic membrane perforation

2. A 29-year-old female presents with complaints of abnormal tastes, difficulty opening her mouth, dry mouth, and facial pain while eating. Physical examination revealed swelling in front of the ears and below the jaw. Based on the patient's history and physical examination, which of the following is the most appropriate diagnosis?
   (A) Parotitis
   (B) Laryngitis
   (C) Epiglottitis
   (D) Pharyngitis
   (E) Oral candidiasis

3. A 40-year-old woman presents with a persistent lump on her wrist. Which of the following is the most appropriate diagnosis?
   (A) Carpal tunnel
   (B) Rheumatoid arthritis
   (C) Ganglion cyst
   (D) Osteoarthritis
   (E) Hematoma

4. A 24-year-old female presents with painful redness, swelling, and pus-filled blisters around the cuticles of the fingernails. Which of the following would be the most appropriate diagnosis?
   (A) Onychomycosis
   (B) Paronychia
   (C) Dermatitis
   (D) Erysipelas
   (E) Impetigo

5. A 28-year-old male presents with several painful open sores on the inside of the mouth and upper throat. Which of the following is the most appropriate diagnosis?
   (A) Oral candidiasis
   (B) Oral leukoplakia
   (C) Aphthous ulcers
   (D) Oral herpes simplex
   (E) Peritonsillar abscess

ANSWER KEY AND EXPLANATIONS

1. D	2. A	3. C	4. B	5. C

1. **The correct answer is (D).** Cholesteatoma is a type of skin cyst located in the middle ear that is primarily caused by recurrent ear infections. Poor function in the eustachian tube leads to negative pressure in the middle ear. This pulls a part of the eardrum into the middle ear, creating a pocket or cyst that fills with old skin cells and other waste material.

2. **The correct answer is (A).** Parotitis is defined as inflammation of the parotid glands, which are the largest of the salivary glands. Parotitis can manifest with abnormal tastes or foul tastes, difficulty opening the mouth, dry mouth, mouth or facial pain while eating, redness on the affected side of the face or neck, and swelling in the front of the ears or behind the jaw.

3. **The correct answer is (C).** A ganglion cyst is a swelling that often occurs at the joints or tendons of the hand or foot. These are most commonly found on the dorsum of the wrist and on the fingers. Ganglion cysts are commonly referred to as bible cysts or bible bumps.

4. **The correct answer is (B).** Paronychia is a skin infection that occurs around the nails. This disorder is most commonly associated with a painful, red, swollen area around the nail, often at the cuticle or at the site of a hangnail or other injury. Pus-filled blisters may also be associated with this condition.

5. **The correct answer is (C).** Aphthous ulcers are also known as canker sores. These ulcers are several painful open sores on the inside of the mouth and upper throat characterized by a break in the mucous membranes.

SUMMING IT UP

- History taking and performing physical examinations questions are intended to evaluate your ability to conduct thorough, focused interviews; recognize important and relevant historical information; perform comprehensive physical examinations; recognize signs, symptoms, and risk factors for selected conditions; and use the data gathered to arrive at a diagnosis.

- To prepare for questions related to this domain, be sure to review the recommended techniques for reviewing and applying historical information, conducting appropriate patient interviews, and performing adequate physical examinations.

- When answering history taking and performing physical examinations questions, be sure to pay attention to the details presented in each question and remember that your overall goal in taking patient histories and performing physical examinations is to arrive at an accurate diagnosis of the patient's medical condition.

CHAPTER 5

Formulating the Most Likely Diagnosis Questions

OVERVIEW

- **Preparing for formulating the most likely diagnosis questions**
- **Tips for answering formulating the most likely diagnosis questions**
- **Practice questions**
- **Answer key and explanations**
- **Summing it up**

PREPARING FOR FORMULATING THE MOST LIKELY DIAGNOSIS QUESTIONS

Formulating the most likely diagnosis questions are another set of questions on the PANRE. The questions pertaining to formulating the most likely diagnosis are designed to test your ability to correctly diagnose a patient based on history, observations, and laboratory and diagnostic studies. This group of questions makes up 18 percent of the exam or about 43 items.

The formulating the most likely diagnosis domain of the PANRE may include questions based on a variety of topics, such as:

- identifying the most likely diagnosis based on available information;
- recognizing the significance of medical history, physical findings, and the results of laboratory and diagnostic studies as they relate to making a diagnosis;
- formulating differential diagnoses; and
- correlating both normal and abnormal diagnostic data.

Formulating the most likely diagnosis is, perhaps, the most important part of a physician assistant's responsibilities. The course of treatment for any patient begins with, and is primarily dictated by, the diagnosis of his or her condition. As a result, being able to make an accurate diagnosis through the use of all available information is a critical skill set for a prospective physician assistant.

Formulating the most likely diagnosis questions will require you to demonstrate your ability to determine the correct diagnosis based on history, observations, and laboratory and diagnostic studies; correlate normal and abnormal diagnostic data; and formulate differential diagnoses.

Most of these questions will, as the name of the domain implies, ask you to identify the correct diagnosis of a given patient's condition. In order to do this, you will have to rely on information you are given about the patient in the question. This information may be related to the patient's medical history, the physical findings you observe during the examination, and/or the results of various laboratory or diagnostic tests. Some of these questions may also require you to arrive at your conclusion by making a differential diagnosis, which means making a diagnosis through a process of elimination.

When you are studying for formulating the most likely diagnosis questions, you should be sure that you are familiar with the signs and symptoms of common conditions and the appropriate methods of diagnosis. You should make certain that you understand the importance of medical history, physical findings, and diagnostic testing results and how to properly use this information to make an accurate diagnosis.

For those questions that ask you to make a differential diagnosis, you should be sure that you have a firm understanding of the process involved in making such a diagnosis.

The multiple-choice questions on the PANRE will require you to choose the correct answer from a field of five choices.

TIPS FOR ANSWERING FORMULATING THE MOST LIKELY DIAGNOSIS QUESTIONS

When you are taking the PANRE, you may find it helpful to remember these hints:

1. Pay close attention to the patient's signs and symptoms. In many cases, the specific signs and symptoms your patient exhibits will be the most important factor in your diagnosis. Be sure to take note of the patient's clinical presentation and keep this information in mind as you consider the possible diagnoses.

2. Take everything into consideration. Though the patient's clinical presentation may be the most important factor to consider, remember to use all the information you have at your disposal. All the data you are given are important and play an important role in determining the correct diagnosis. Pay attention to all of the details in each question.

3. Be efficient. The PANRE is a closely timed examination, so you only have a short amount of time to spend on each question. Though you will want to read carefully and pay close attention to the details, you will need to do so quickly. Try scanning the question and eliminating any obviously incorrect answer choices. This can help you to focus your concentration on the important elements of the question and arrive at an answer more quickly.

PRACTICE QUESTIONS

Directions: Choose the option that best answers the question.

1. A 24-year-old male presents after a motor vehicle accident with blood accumulation filling over 1/2 of the space of the anterior chamber of the right eye. Which of the following is the most accurate diagnosis?
   (A) Hordeolum
   (B) Orbital cellulitis
   (C) Hyphema
   (D) Nystagmus
   (E) Pterygium

2. A 52-year-old postmenopausal woman presents with urine leakage when coughing or sneezing as well as incomplete emptying of the bladder. Which of the following is the most appropriate diagnosis?
   (A) Vaginitis
   (B) Cystitis
   (C) Cystocele
   (D) Rectocele
   (E) Vaginal prolapse

3. A 60-year-old female, with a previous history of hysterectomy, presents with vaginal pressure, painful intercourse, constipation, and intermittent vaginal bleeding. Which of the following is the most appropriate diagnosis?
   (A) Vaginitis
   (B) Cystitis
   (C) Cystocele
   (D) Rectocele
   (E) Vaginal prolapse

4. An 8-year-old boy presents with involuntary, excessive eye blinking, facial grimacing, and shoulder shrugging. In addition, he also has been noticed muttering inappropriate words and repeating words or phrases he hears from other people. Which of the following is the most appropriate diagnosis?
   (A) Huntingdon's disease
   (B) Parkinson's disease
   (C) Guillain-Barre syndrome
   (D) Attention deficit disorder
   (E) Tourette syndrome

5. A 32-year-old woman, who has never been pregnant, presents with inappropriate and spontaneous flow of milk from her breasts. Which of the following is the most appropriate diagnosis?
   (A) Mastitis
   (B) Galactorrhea
   (C) Gynecomastia
   (D) Fibrocystic disease
   (E) Breast abscess

ANSWER KEY AND EXPLANATIONS

1. C	2. C	3. D	4. E	5. B

1. **The correct answer is (C).** Hyphema, by definition, is blood accumulation in the front part of the eye. This disorder is most often caused by trauma to the eye; however, hyphema can also be caused by cancer of the eye, blood vessel abnormalities of the eye, and inflammation of the iris.

2. **The correct answer is (C).** A cystocele, otherwise known as a fallen bladder, occurs when the wall between a woman's bladder and her vagina weakens and allows the bladder to droop into the vagina. This condition may cause unwanted urine leakage when coughing, sneezing, or laughing as well as incomplete emptying of the bladder.

3. **The correct answer is (D).** A rectocele is a tear in the rectovaginal septum. The two causes of this disorder are childbirth and hysterectomy. Individuals with a rectocele may experience vaginal pressure, painful intercourse, constipation, intermittent vaginal bleeding, difficulty passing stools, incomplete emptying of the colon, and a feeling of something "falling" from the vagina.

4. **The correct answer is (E).** Tourette syndrome is a neurological disorder characterized by repetitive, stereotyped, involuntary movements and vocalizations called tics. Individuals with this disorder can experience excessive eye blinking, facial grimacing, and shoulder shrugging. In addition, this disorder may result in muttering inappropriate words or profanity and repeating words or phrases heard from other people.

5. **The correct answer is (B).** Galactorrhea is defined as the inappropriate and spontaneous flow of milk from the breasts that is not associated with pregnancy, childbirth, and nursing. This condition will affect 20–25 percent of the female population at one time or another and, although rare, can also occur in males.

SUMMING IT UP

- Formulating the most likely diagnosis questions will require an understanding of the importance of patient medical history, physical findings, and the results of laboratory and diagnostic studies to the formation of a diagnosis and of the methods involved in forming a differential diagnosis.

- When you are studying for formulating the most likely diagnosis questions, be sure to familiarize yourself with the various signs and symptoms of common medical conditions. You should also make sure that you know how to use other information, such as medical history and data obtained from diagnostic testing, to establish a diagnosis.

- Pay attention to the details in each question. Since your diagnosis is entirely based on the information provided to you in the question, it is critically important that you pay close attention to this data. These details will offer you important clues that can steer you toward the correct answer. Take everything into consideration and make your choice carefully.

CHAPTER 6

Health Maintenance Questions

OVERVIEW

- **Preparing for health maintenance questions**
- **Tips for answering health maintenance questions**
- **Practice questions**
- **Answer key and explanations**
- **Summing it up**

PREPARING FOR HEALTH MAINTENANCE QUESTIONS

Health maintenance questions are a fourth subgroup of questions on the PANRE. The questions pertaining to health maintenance will test your knowledge of a wide variety of topics related to disease prevention and the overall maintenance of good health. This group of questions makes up 10 percent of the exam or about 24 items.

The health maintenance domain of the PANRE may include questions based on a variety of topics, such as:

- adapting various health maintenance techniques to a patient's specific needs;
- communicating effectively with patients about health maintenance;
- using counseling, patient education techniques, and informational databases;
- epidemiology of given conditions;
- prevention and early detection of given conditions;
- the relative value of routine screening tests;
- patient education regarding preventable diseases or lifestyle changes;
- healthy lifestyles;
- communicable disease prevention;
- immunization schedules and recommendations;
- the risks and benefits associated with immunization;
- growth and development;
- sexuality;
- risks associated with environmental or occupational exposure;

- the effects of stress;

- the psychological impact of disease or injury;

- aging;

- indications of abuse or neglect; and

- barriers to proper care.

The practice of medicine isn't just about diagnosing and treating diseases. It's also about preventing them. As a physician assistant, you must be familiar with the common methods of disease prevention, the risk factors associated with various diseases, the impact of a patient's daily life on his or her health, and the many ways to promote long-term good health.

Health maintenance questions are designed to test your ability to adapt various health maintenance techniques to a patient's specific needs; communicate effectively with patients about health maintenance; and use counseling, patient education techniques, and informational databases to facilitate health maintenance.

The multiple-choice questions on the PANRE will require you to choose the correct answer from a field of five choices.

TIPS FOR ANSWERING HEALTH MAINTENANCE QUESTIONS

When you are taking the PANRE, you may find it helpful to remember these hints:

1. Remember what you have learned. The health maintenance domain covers a broad range of topics, many of which are closely tied to other domains. Referencing the information you have used to study for other portions of the PANRE may be helpful when answering health maintenance questions.

2. Think critically. Some of these questions may ask you to choose the best course of action in a given situation. When you encounter such a question, read the scenario carefully, examine your options, and quickly think about the pros and cons of each before you make a selection.

3. Pay close attention to details. As with any question on the PANRE, make sure you pay attention to all of the details provided and take them all into consideration before proceeding. You will need to know as much about the scenario in each question as possible in order to choose the correct answer.

PRACTICE QUESTIONS

1. Hypertriglyceridemia can effectively be managed with daily consumption of which of the following vitamins?
   (A) Niacin
   (B) Vitamin C
   (C) Vitamin D
   (D) Riboflavin
   (E) Thiamine

2. Individuals who suffer from phenylketonuria should avoid a diet rich in which of the following substances?
   (A) Sugar
   (B) Fat
   (C) Salt
   (D) Protein
   (E) Carbohydrates

3. Fecal impaction may result from overuse of which of the following over-the-counter medications?
   (A) Antacids
   (B) Fever reducers
   (C) NSAIDS
   (D) Laxatives
   (E) Cough suppressants

4. Methimazole is commonly prescribed for maintenance treatment of which of the following disorders?
   (A) Hyperparathyroidism
   (B) Hypoparathyroidism
   (C) Hyperthyroidism
   (D) Hypothyroidism
   (E) Subacute thyroiditis

5. Gout can result from an accumulation of _____ in joints.
   (A) Folic acid
   (B) Citric acid
   (C) Uric acid
   (D) Omega-3 fatty acids
   (E) Omega-6 fatty acids

ANSWER KEY AND EXPLANATIONS

1. A	2. D	3. A	4. C	5. C

1. **The correct answer is (A).** The B-complex vitamin, niacin, has been proven clinically effective for treatment of hypertriglyceridemia. Administration of at least 1.5 grams/day can reduce triglyceride levels by up to 50 percent.

2. **The correct answer is (D).** Individuals with phenylketonuria should avoid foods rich in phenylalanine, which is contained primarily in protein-rich foods such as fish, chicken, milk, cheese, and eggs.

3. **The correct answer is (A).** Overuse of antacids, particularly antacids that contain aluminum, can result in constipation that progresses to the point of fecal impaction. Other medications that may cause fecal impaction include calcium channel blockers, antidepressants, and tranquilizers.

4. **The correct answer is (C).** Methimazole, more commonly referred to as Tapazole, is used to treat hyperthyroidism, a condition that occurs when the thyroid gland produces too much thyroid hormone.

5. **The correct answer is (C).** Gout occurs when high levels of uric acid in the blood cause crystals to form and accumulate around a joint. A diet with reduced amounts of red meat, dairy products, alcohol, and sugar should reduce the amount of uric acid and assist in relieving gout symptoms.

SUMMING IT UP

- The health maintenance questions on the PANRE are designed to test your abilities with regard to adapting various health maintenance techniques to a patient's specific needs; communicating effectively with patients about health maintenance; and using counseling, patient education techniques, and informational databases to facilitate health maintenance.

- The topics covered in this domain include the epidemiology of given conditions, prevention and early detection of given conditions, the relative value of routine screening tests, patient education regarding preventable diseases or lifestyle changes, healthy lifestyles, communicable disease prevention, immunization schedules and recommendations, the risks and benefits associated with immunization, growth and development, sexuality, risks associated with environmental or occupational exposure, the effects of stress, the psychological impact of disease or injury, aging, indications of abuse or neglect, and barriers to proper care.

CHAPTER 7

Clinical Intervention Questions

OVERVIEW

- **Preparing for clinical intervention questions**
- **Tips for answering clinical intervention questions**
- **Practice questions**
- **Answer key and explanations**
- **Summing it up**

PREPARING FOR CLINICAL INTERVENTION QUESTIONS

Clinical intervention questions are a fifth type of question you will encounter on the PANRE. The questions pertaining to clinical intervention will test your knowledge of a wide variety of issues related to the overall process of care. This group of questions makes up 14 percent of the exam or about 34 items.

The clinical intervention domain of the PANRE may include questions based on a variety of topics, such as:

- the formation and implementation of treatment plans;
- your ability to demonstrate expertise in performing various procedures;
- using effective methods of communication and counseling techniques;
- encouraging patient participation in and adherence to treatment plans;
- treating selected medical conditions;
- the indications, contraindications, benefits, risks, potential complications, and techniques for certain procedures;
- standard precautions;
- special isolation procedures;
- sterilization techniques;
- monitoring therapeutic regiments;
- recognizing medical emergencies;
- hospital admissions and discharges;
- community resources;
- patient education;

- working with other medical professionals;

- end-of-life concerns; and

- the potential benefits and risks of alternative medicine.

Clinical intervention is a very broad topic that covers a large portion of the regular responsibilities of a physician assistant. Having a firm understanding of various clinical intervention techniques and procedures is essential for the physician assistant.

Clinical intervention questions on the PANRE are designed to test your skills as they relate to concepts like the formation and implementation of treatment plans, your ability to demonstrate expertise in performing various procedures, using effective methods of communication and counseling techniques, and encouraging patient participation in and adherence to treatment plans.

When you prepare for clinical intervention questions, you should focus on building a firm understanding of the fundamental principles underlying the basic process of care. Reviewing the concepts and topics mentioned above will go a long way toward ensuring that you are ready for both the clinical intervention domain and the rest of the PANRE.

The multiple-choice questions on the PANRE will require you to choose the correct answer from a field of five choices.

TIPS FOR ANSWERING CLINICAL INTERVENTION QUESTIONS

When you are taking the PANRE, you may find it helpful to remember these hints:

1. Use what you already know. Since clinical intervention questions are frequently related to topics covered in other domains, use what you have learned while studying for these other domains to help you choose the correct answer. Being well prepared for the other parts of the PANRE will be very helpful when it comes to answering clinical intervention questions.

2. Pay close attention to the details. As with many questions on the PANRE, the details included in clinical intervention questions are critically important. Be sure to take all the details into consideration before making a choice. Ignoring or overlooking details may lead you to an incorrect solution.

3. Be efficient. The PANRE is a closely timed examination, so you only have a short amount of time to spend on each question. Though you will want to read carefully and pay close attention to the details, you will need to do so quickly. Try scanning the question and eliminating any obviously incorrect answer choices. This can help you to focus your concentration on the important elements of the question and arrive at an answer more quickly.

PRACTICE QUESTIONS

1. An 80-year-old female presents with sick sinus syndrome. Which of the following procedures are required to treat this condition?
   (A) Cardiac catheterization
   (B) Coronary artery bypass graft
   (C) Cardiac ablation
   (D) Pacemaker insertion
   (E) Coronary stenting

2. Which of the following is the proper intervention when individuals with thrombotic thrombocytopenic purpura are unresponsive to treatments?
   (A) Plasmapheresis
   (B) Splenectomy
   (C) Intravenous anticoagulants
   (D) Intravenous antibiotics
   (E) High-dose corticosteroids

3. Orchiopexy is the surgical procedure performed in order to correct which of the following disorders?
   (A) Testicular torsion
   (B) Epididymitis
   (C) Hydrocele
   (D) Cryptorchidism
   (E) Orchitis

4. Which of the following types of medications is an appropriate intervention for a seizure lasting longer than 30 minutes?
   (A) Benzodiazepines
   (B) Imidazopyridines
   (C) Pyrazolopyrimidines
   (D) Cyclopyrrolones
   (E) b-Carbolines

5. Intravenous Amphotericin B combined with oral flucytosine has been proven to be an effective treatment for which of the following infectious diseases?
   (A) Malaria
   (B) Cryptococcosis
   (C) Shigellosis
   (D) Salmonellosis
   (E) Botulism

ANSWER KEY AND EXPLANATIONS

1. D	2. B	3. D	4. A	5. B

1. **The correct answer is (D).** Sick sinus syndrome is a disorder characterized by malfunction of the sinus node, the heart's primary pacemaker. This disorder can cause abnormal and dangerously slow heart rates. It is primarily treated by the placement of a pacemaker.

2. **The correct answer is (B).** Thrombotic thrombocytopenic purpura is a blood disorder that causes blood clots to form in small blood vessels around the body. This leads to a low platelet count. Individuals who are unresponsive to treatments or have several recurrences should undergo a splenectomy to correct this disorder.

3. **The correct answer is (D).** Cryptorchidism is a disorder of an undescended testicle. Orchiopexy is performed to move an undescended testicle into the scrotum and permanently fix it there.

4. **The correct answer is (A).** Seizures that last for longer than 30 minutes are characteristic of the disorder of status epilepticus. Randomized controlled trials show that benzodiazepines, particularly diazepam and lorazepam, should be the initial drug therapy in patients with status epilepticus.

5. **The correct answer is (B).** Cryptococcosis is a potentially fatal fungal disease that is particularly damaging to individuals with weakened immune systems, such as HIV patients. Intravenous Amphotericin B combined with oral flucytosine has been proven to be an effective treatment for this disorder, and this medical intervention does not further weaken the immune system.

SUMMING IT UP

- The clinical intervention domain is designed to test your knowledge of a wide variety of issues related to the overall process of care.

- Clinical intervention questions will be based on a broad range of topics, including the formation and implementation of treatment plans; your ability to demonstrate expertise in performing various procedures; using effective methods of communication and counseling techniques, including encouraging patient participation in and adherence to treatment plans; managing and treating selected medical conditions and monitoring therapeutic regimens; the indications, contraindications, benefits, risks, potential complications, and techniques for certain procedures; standard precautions as well as special isolation measures and sterilization techniques; recognizing medical emergencies; hospital admissions and discharges; community resources; patient education; working with other medical professionals; end-of-life concerns; and the potential benefits and risks of alternative medicine.

- Many of these questions are related to other PANRE domains, so a firm understanding of the other topics covered on the test will likely improve your performance on this section.

CHAPTER 8

Pharmaceutical Therapeutics Questions

OVERVIEW

- Preparing for pharmaceutical therapeutics questions
- Tips for answering pharmaceutical therapeutics questions
- Practice questions
- Answer key and explanations
- Summing it up

PREPARING FOR PHARMACEUTICAL THERAPEUTICS QUESTIONS

Pharmaceutical therapeutics questions are a sixth category of questions on the PANRE. The questions pertaining to pharmaceutical therapeutics are designed to test your knowledge of the vast array of drugs administered by physician assistants and your ability to use them properly. This group of questions makes up 18 percent of the exam or about 43 items.

The pharmaceutical therapeutics domain of the PANRE is comprised of questions based on many different topics, including:

- choosing the best pharmacologic treatment for a specific condition;
- mechanism of action;
- indications and contraindications for use;
- possible side effects;
- potential adverse reactions;
- monitoring and follow-up of pharmacologic regimens;
- risks related to drug interactions;
- clinical presentation and treatment of drug interactions;
- drug toxicity;
- cross reactivity;
- methods used to reduce medication errors; and
- recognizing and treating allergic reactions.

Pharmaceutical therapeutics, which refers to the prescription and administration of drugs to treat a specific medical condition, is a very important part of the job of a physician assistant. In most cases, physician assistants are authorized to prescribe, dispense, and administer a wide variety of drugs. As such, it is extremely important that any current or prospective physician assistant has a firm understanding of the many different types of drugs he or she will encounter in the course of practice.

Pharmaceutical therapeutics questions on the PANRE will ask about choosing the most appropriate pharmaceutical treatment for a given condition; monitoring and adjusting pharmacological regimens as needed; and recognizing, evaluating, and properly reporting adverse reactions.

Some questions may require you to recognize the mechanism of action of a particular drug, the indications and contraindications for its use, the possible side effects, potential adverse reactions, the risks for and presentation and treatment of drug interactions, drug toxicity, the cross-reactivity of similar drugs, and the methods used to reduce medication errors.

The PANRE also includes questions that are designed to test your ability to monitor and evaluate a patient's pharmacological regimen. These questions will require you to have a strong understanding of potential drug interactions and how to recognize and treat any complications that may arise from such interactions. You will also need to demonstrate your ability to recognize and treat allergic reactions.

The multiple-choice questions on the PANRE will require you to choose the correct answer from a field of five choices.

TIPS FOR ANSWERING PHARMACEUTICAL THERAPEUTICS QUESTIONS

When you are taking the PANRE, you may find it helpful to remember these hints:

1. The right drug for one patient may not be the right drug for all patients. Every patient is different. The effect a certain drug has on one patient may be significantly different from the effect it has on another. When you are asked to choose the most appropriate drug to administer to a given patient, be sure to pay close attention to the specific information you are given about that patient's condition and history. Though there are general guidelines for prescribing and administering drugs that you should routinely follow, you must be sure to adjust your approach based on the particular circumstances of the given situation.

2. Many drugs have multiple applications. Many of the drugs you will need to be familiar with can be used in more than one way. Remember that a certain drug may have alternative uses beyond its main purpose. When you are considering which medication you should prescribe, keep these additional uses in mind.

3. Remember when a drug should or should not be used. Remembering to consider the indications and contraindications for using a particular drug is critically important. When you are faced with choosing the best drug to use, remember to pay close attention to the specifics of the patient's condition and his or her presenting signs and symptoms. The patient's signs and symptoms may indicate or contraindicate the use of a certain medication. Be sure that the drug you choose is appropriate for the patient at hand.

4. Be sure you're familiar with the following drug classifications:

- Analgesics and anti-inflammatory drugs
- Anesthetics
- Antidotes and reversal agents

- Antimicrobials
- Antiparasitic drugs
- Cardiovascular drugs
- Chemotherapeutic and immunological drugs

- Gastrointestinal drugs
- Hormones and other endocrine drugs
- Respiratory drugs
- Topical drugs

PRACTICE QUESTIONS

1. Which of the following is an appropriate treatment for oral candidiasis?
   (A) Cipro
   (B) Nystatin
   (C) Ampicillin
   (D) Levaquin
   (E) Zithromax

2. Which of the following anti-inflammatory medications is commonly used in conjunction with ibuprofen for treatment of acute pericarditis?
   (A) Colchicine
   (B) Naproxen
   (C) Azapropazone
   (D) Etodolac
   (E) Meloxicam

3. Helminth infections are most effectively treated by which of the following medications?
   (A) Combantrin
   (B) Mebendazole
   (C) Abamectin
   (D) Ivermectin
   (E) Triclabendazole

4. The dermatologic condition of alopecia is commonly treated by which of the following medications?
   (A) Erythromycin
   (B) Clindamycin
   (C) Minoxidil
   (D) Accutane
   (E) Tretinoin

5. Birth-control pills can prevent the occurrence of which of the following disorders?
   (A) Cystocele
   (B) Rectocele
   (C) Ovarian tumors
   (D) Ovarian cysts
   (E) Cervical tumors

ANSWER KEY AND EXPLANATIONS

1. B	2. A	3. A	4. C	5. D

1. **The correct answer is (B).** Oral candidiasis is an infection of the mucous membranes of the mouth that is caused by yeast fungi. Nystatin is an anti-fungal medication that is useful for treatment of this disorder. The other four medications on the list are antibacterial medications.

2. **The correct answer is (A).** Colchicine is an older and well-established anti-inflammatory drug that can help control the inflammation and prevent pericarditis from recurring weeks or even months later. Sometimes, colchicine is used in conjunction with NSAIDs, e.g., ibuprofen.

3. **The correct answer is (A).** Helminth infections are caused by a parasitic worm that infests the body. Combantrin is the drug of choice for treating this type of infection due to the fact that it paralyzes the worms, preventing them from attaching to the walls of the intestines.

4. **The correct answer is (C).** Alopecia is the disorder of thinning hair or hair loss either in a pattern or in spots. Minoxidil, commonly known as Rogaine, is the most effective medication to stop hair loss and promote hair growth.

5. **The correct answer is (D).** Birth-control pills may be very effective in preventing further occurrences of ovarian cysts. In addition, birth-control pills can also greatly reduce the risk of developing ovarian cancer.

SUMMING IT UP

- Pharmaceutical therapeutics questions will require you to demonstrate your ability to choose the most appropriate pharmaceutical treatment for a given condition; monitor and adjust pharmacological regimens as needed; and recognize, evaluate, and properly report adverse reactions.

- When preparing for pharmaceutical therapeutics questions, you will need to be sure that you are keenly familiar with the various drugs used in the field of medicine. Remember to pay close attention to the mechanism of action, indications and contraindications for use, side effects, potential adverse reactions, drug interactions, drug toxicity, and cross-reactivity. You should also be sure that you are able to recognize and treat any potential reactions or interactions and are familiar with the methods for reducing medication errors.

- Read the details of the questions carefully. The information the questions provide concerning the patient's condition, especially his or her signs and symptoms, will play a crucial role in determining the best course of action. Pay close attention to these details and remember to keep in mind the indications, contraindications, and alternative uses of the drugs you are considering.

CHAPTER 9

Applying Basic Science Concepts Questions

OVERVIEW

- **Preparing for applying basic science concepts questions**
- **Tips for answering applying basic science concepts questions**
- **Practice questions**
- **Answer key and explanations**
- **Summing it up**

PREPARING FOR APPLYING BASIC SCIENCE CONCEPTS QUESTIONS

Applying basic science concepts questions are the final type of question on the PANRE. The questions pertaining to applying basic science concepts will test your knowledge of the basic scientific principles related to human health and the diagnosis of medical conditions. This group of questions makes up 10 percent of the exam or about 24 items.

The applying basic science concepts domain of the PANRE may include questions based on a variety of topics, such as:

- anatomy, physiology, pathophysiology, microbiology, and biochemistry;
- the pathological process of disease;
- identifying normal and abnormal anatomy and physiology;
- relating pathophysiologic principles to selected disease processes;
- relating abnormal physical examination findings to selected disease processes; and
- relating abnormal diagnostic testing results to selected disease processes.

The practice of medicine is based on the fundamental principles of a wide array of sciences, including biology, chemistry, physiology, and anatomy, among others. For physician assistants, or any medical professionals, having a solid understanding of the basic science behind medicine is critically important. The ability to appropriately and accurately examine, diagnose, and treat patients is founded on a strong scientific understanding of the human body, health, and disease.

Applying basic science concepts questions will require you to have a basic understanding of the various sciences related to the practice of medicine. Most notably, you will need to be familiar with basic principles of human anatomy and physiology, pathophysiology, microbiology, and biochemistry.

Applying basic science concepts questions are designed to test your ability to identify normal and abnormal anatomy and physiology and relate pathophysiologic principles, abnormal physical examination findings, and abnormal diagnostic testing results to selected disease processes.

One of the most important concepts to review in preparation for applying basic science concepts questions is the pathological process of disease. The pathological process of a given disease includes its cause (often called its etiology), its mechanism of development (or pathogenesis), the changes it causes, and the effects it eventually has on a patient. Many of the questions in this domain will be focused on or related to pathological processes in some way.

When you study for the applying basic science concepts domain, be sure to familiarize yourself with the basic principles of the important sciences associated with the practice of medicine. You should also be sure to develop a broad understanding of the pathological process of disease, both as a concept and as it applies to various common medical conditions.

The multiple-choice questions on the PANRE will require you to choose the correct answer from a field of five choices.

TIPS FOR ANSWERING APPLYING BASIC SCIENCE CONCEPTS QUESTIONS

When you are taking the PANRE, you may find it helpful to remember these hints:

1. Remember what you have learned. This portion of the PANRE is primarily based on hard science, so you will likely have to rely on the specific information you have studied in order to arrive at the correct answer. However, since the concepts covered in this domain ultimately inform every aspect of the practice of medicine, it may also be helpful to keep the information you have learned while studying for other domains in mind as well.

2. Pay close attention to details. As with all of the other domains on the PANRE, it is very important to pay close attention to the details included in the applying basic science concepts questions. Make sure you understand exactly what the question is asking and remember to take all the provided details into consideration.

PRACTICE QUESTIONS

1. Exanthem is defined as a widespread rash caused by a virus or bacteria that normally occurs in children. Which of the following types of exanthem is caused by a bacterium?
   (A) Measles
   (B) Mumps
   (C) Erythema infectiosum
   (D) Scarlet fever
   (E) Roseola infantum

2. Condyloma acuminatum is a dermatologic disorder caused by which of the following viruses?
   (A) HIV virus
   (B) Human papilloma virus
   (C) Human parainfluenza virus
   (D) Varicella zoster virus
   (E) Parvovirus

3. Which of the following refers to an abnormal or difficult pregnancy or childbirth that is often assisted by forceps, ventouse, or caesarian section?
   (A) Dystocia
   (B) Ectopic pregnancy
   (C) Abruptio placentae
   (D) Spontaneous abortion
   (E) Placenta previa

4. Which of the following types of bacteria is the most common cause of bullous impetigo?
   (A) *Staphylococcus epidermis*
   (B) *Staphylococcus folliculitis*
   (C) *Staphylococcus saprophyticus*
   (D) *Staphylococcus aureus*
   (E) *Staphylococcus hominis*

5. Individuals who are diagnosed with G6PD deficiency are susceptible to which of the following types of anemia?
   (A) Iron-deficiency anemia
   (B) Pernicious anemia
   (C) Hemolytic anemia
   (D) Sickle cell anemia
   (E) Folate-deficiency anemia

ANSWER KEY AND EXPLANATIONS

1. D	2. B	3. A	4. D	5. C

1. **The correct answer is (D).** Scarlet fever is a form of exanthem that is caused by the *Streptococcus pyogenes* bacteria. Measles, mumps, erythema infectiosum, and roseola infantum are all exanthems that are caused by viruses.

2. **The correct answer is (B).** Condyloma acuminatum, commonly known as genital warts, is a dermatologic disorder caused by the human papilloma virus.

3. **The correct answer is (A).** Dystocia is defined as abnormal or difficult pregnancy or childbirth. Approximately one out of every five childbirths involves dystocia. Dystocia is caused by incoordinate uterine activity, abnormal fetal lie, or presentation. These childbirths are assisted by forceps, ventouse, or caesarian section.

4. **The correct answer is (D).** Impetigo is a contagious skin infection that usually produces blisters or sores on the face, neck, hands, and diaper area and is one of the most common skin infections among children. Bullous impetigo, the form that produces large blisters, is most commonly caused by the *Staphylococcus aureus* bacteria.

5. **The correct answer is (C).** G6PD deficiency is an inherited condition in which the body doesn't have enough of the enzyme glucose-6-phosphate dehydrogenase, or G6PD, which helps red blood cells function normally. This deficiency can cause hemolytic anemia.

SUMMING IT UP

- The applying basic science concepts questions on the PANRE focus on the basic scientific principles associated with the practice of medicine. Some of the sciences that will be involved in these questions include human anatomy and physiology, pathophysiology, microbiology, and biochemistry.

- The applying basic science concepts questions are designed to test your ability to identify normal and abnormal anatomy and physiology and relate pathophysiologic principles, abnormal physical examination findings, and abnormal diagnostic testing results to selected disease processes.

PART III

STUDY GUIDE

CHAPTER 10

How to Prepare for the PANRE

HOW TO STUDY FOR THE TEST

When to Start Studying for the PANRE

Well before the actual test date, you should develop a study plan to begin reviewing for the PANRE. Since effective preparation for the exam can range from several months to a full year, start thinking in advance about how you can direct your reading and learning, as well as your clinical activities, to passing the exam. Schedule frequent reviews of medical and surgical concepts covered on the PANRE's content blueprint and resist the urge to cram this information into last-minute study sessions. As you undoubtedly learned in college, cramming is not a successful test-taking strategy since it is difficult to retain large amounts of information in a short time. Moreover, staying up late the night before the exam will only leave you feeling overwhelmed and exhausted on your test date. Generally speaking, it is better to schedule multiple review periods over a longer period of time instead of trying to review all of your notes and study guides shortly before your test date. Frequent studying for shorter blocks of time over the course of several months will ensure greater retention and allow you to thoroughly master the information before you take the PANRE.

Strategies for Effective Test Preparation

As you begin to study for the PANRE, it may be helpful to consider a few test-taking strategies that will allow you to approach the exam feeling confident and well-prepared:

- Ask yourself questions as you read over your notes and other study materials pertaining to medical and surgical concepts you find to be the most challenging. By answering further questions about difficult material, you are reinforcing your knowledge and discovering areas where more intensive study is needed. It may be useful to predict and answer potential exam questions to pinpoint which topics you've learned well and which ones need more review.

- Target your exam review to subject areas outside of your clinical activity. Physician assistants working in the area of primary care may not have to prepare quite as much for generalist questions as those working in a particular specialty since they review these concepts at work on a daily basis. If you are not currently practicing as a PA-C, you will probably need to spend more time reviewing medical and surgical concepts to refresh your memory and prepare for the exam.

- Focus your continuing medical education (CME) hours on primary care or an area that is not part of your current practice or expertise. This strategy will help you learn and remember concepts that you otherwise might not encounter or have a chance to review frequently and help you increase your knowledge related to those areas for the exam.

- Review sample questions for the PANRE several months before the exam. Using study guides like this book, start looking over typical test questions and take practice exams to get an idea about the types of questions that will be asked and the scope of the material being covered. You will find a diagnostic test and two full-length practice tests in this book. When taking these tests, try to simulate the actual test-taking situation by eliminating distractions and tracking the amount of time it takes you to complete a full-length test. If you find that you are exceeding the 240 total minutes you are allotted for the PANRE, brainstorm methods for improving your time, such as spending less time on questions you do not know and dedicating more study time to the difficult topics you encounter during the practice tests. Taking practice exams will allow you to target any areas of weakness you might identify and help you decide how to spend your remaining review time most productively to strengthen your knowledge base in those particular areas. The more you practice before taking the PANRE, the less anxiety you will experience on test day.

- Form a study group. Group learning allows each member to benefit from the knowledge of others in the group and is especially helpful for those who learn best through verbal exchanges of information, including speaking and conversation. Your group may prefer to review a specific organ system each time you meet, for example, or each group member could research and develop questions related to a particular task area to help the other group members retain the information.

- Create note cards. For students who learn well by writing or typing facts, this tried-and-true study method can be very helpful. Creating note cards may help you to remember information for an exam by taking larger concepts and narrowing them down to smaller, more concise thoughts that may be written or typed and then memorized. To study for the PANRE, for example, you could make a group of note cards for each organ system and create individual cards for diseases, disorders, and diagnoses within each system. Using note cards to review for the exam allows you study by yourself without having to schedule time with members of a study group; additionally, you can review note cards frequently whenever you have a few spare moments to reinforce your learning.

- Review your lecture notes and course textbooks. By rereading the material in your course textbooks and studying the accompanying lecture notes from your physician assistant education program, you will recall the information you previously learned in school and reinforce the knowledge and skills you have gained through clinical practice. Some students find that making outlines helps them to organize and manage the information, making it easier to remember these concepts while taking the exam.

- Use pictures and diagrams if you are a visual learner. By drawing, labeling, or creating diagrams for medical information such as organ systems and processes, these concepts will be easier to recall during the exam. It may also help you to color- code study materials to help you process and remember this information using visual cues.

- Allow plenty of time to prepare for your exam. The PANRE is designed to assess the knowledge and skills a certified physician assistant has gained during the six-year certification maintenance cycle. Be sure to reserve adequate time to review the knowledge and skills you have gained in clinical practice as well as the medical and surgical concepts that you learned in your PA education program. It is a good idea to start preparing for the exam at least several months in advance and to practice answering PANRE-style questions. By starting your review early, you can engage in frequent, shorter study sessions over a long period of time and avoid potentially stressful, last-minute study sessions right before the exam.

- Take good care of yourself on a daily basis. To ensure that you are healthy both mentally and physically for the exam, be sure to get plenty of sleep, eat well, and stay hydrated.

TEST-TAKING TIPS FOR THE PANRE: EXAM DAY

On the day of your exam, you will want to be as refreshed, alert, and self-assured with the knowledge that you are as well-prepared as possible. Taking a test can be a stressful experience. The best way to alleviate this stress is to study for the exam well in advance and use the knowledge that you are ready to take the PANRE to bolster your confidence level. Some additional tips for doing your very best on the exam when your test day arrives are included in this section.

Before the Exam Begins

- Be sure to get a good night's rest the night before your exam so you feel your best and can focus on doing your very best work. Getting a full eight hours of sleep the night before your test will leave you feeling refreshed and able to think clearly. Although it might seem like a good idea, do not take any sleep-inducing medications the night before taking the PANRE since you might feel groggy and sluggish the next day.

- Eat a balanced, nutritious meal before taking your exam. Enjoying a healthy meal before taking the PANRE will make you more alert for the test and help to ensure that you are not distracted by hunger during the exam. Good food choices to help you stay full for the duration of your exam include fresh fruits, vegetables, eggs, and fish.

- Avoid drinking too much caffeine on the day of your exam, including coffee or energy drinks. Although caffeinated beverages may give you a quick burst of energy, they may add to your anxiety level or make it more difficult to concentrate. You should also stay away from alcohol the night before the test to avoid dehydration and fatigue the next day. Drinking water or fruit juice will help you to stay refreshed and hydrated on your test day.

- Resist the temptation to conduct an intensive review the night before the exam. It will only be counterproductive to engage in a long, last-minute cramming session the night before your test date. Material you review in this type of study session is usually forgotten since it does not become part of your long-term memory, and trying to cram the night before the exam will only leave you feeling tired the next day. A better idea would be to accept that you have finished studying for the test and find a relaxing activity to enjoy, such as seeing a movie, spending quiet time with family or friends, or reading a book.

- Gather needed items for your test day. Since a chaotic rush the morning of the test will only add to feelings of stress before the exam, take the time to gather what you need the evening before your test. Remember to bring two forms of identification (ID) to the testing center. One of the two IDs must contain a permanently affixed photo with your name and signature. The other should show your printed name and signature. The names on both forms of ID must match your name as it is registered with NCCPA; otherwise, you will not be admitted to the testing center to take the PANRE.

During the Exam

- Before you begin the exam, make sure you understand and review all test directions.

- Do not worry about your performance on the exam. Keep in mind that you have been studying for the PANRE over the course of several years, including your physician assistant education program, your years of continuing medical education (CME), and your experience in clinical practice. All of your accumulated knowledge and skills, in addition to your exam preparation, will serve you well and should allow you to achieve a high score on the PANRE. Instead of worrying, concentrate on the exam"s content and allow yourself to feel confident about doing well on the PANRE.

- Read each question carefully and be sure you understand what is being asked since some questions are more complicated than others. Many questions on the PANRE begin with a "stem" which that poses a typical situation physician assistants might encounter. Be sure you thoroughly comprehend the stem before proceeding to answer the related test questions.

- Answer the questions to the best of your knowledge and realize that test questions are written to be straight-forward. The NCCPA is interested in testing and assessing your knowledge and skills; they do not write trick questions or provide hidden clues.

- Pace yourself within each test block and give your full attention to each question. There is no need to rush since you will have 60 seconds to complete each test question. Most test-takers do not need all the time allotted for each test block, so running out of time is unlikely.

- Review your answer choices carefully as you complete each exam block to ensure that you have answered all the questions to the best of your knowledge and haven't inadvertently skipped any questions.

- Anticipate the answer before selecting your response. As you read the test question, try to decide in advance what the correct answer should be. Then look over the answer choices to see if any of them match your preliminary answer. Read all the available answers and think carefully before you select the best choice. If you find your antici-pated answer in one of the possible choices, be sure to select it. You may also eliminate possible choices using logic and general knowledge if you are unsure of the answer. Then choose an answer from the remaining possibilities.

- Visualize the correct answer to difficult questions. For situational question, it may be helpful to visualize a patient who is in the situation posed by the test question. Thinking about a real-life scenario that involves an actual patient may make an abstract test question seem more concrete and the correct answer to it more logical.

- Expect the exam to focus on general concepts as opposed to atypical medical conditions. The PANRE tends to emphasize commonly seen diseases, disorders, and diagnoses that would not be unusual in a physician assistant"s practice, instead of more rare occurrences. When in doubt, look for the general answer over the exceptional one.

- Notice patterns between question choices and previously learned information. Look for trends and patterns in graphs, tables, and charts, and recognize relationships between test questions and your knowledge base as a physician assistant.

- Think about the intent of the test question. For especially difficult questions, try to assess what type of knowledge the question is trying to gauge or which skill it is trying to test. For example, is the question trying to determine if you can recognize the general symptoms of an illness or is it asking you to diagnose a less-common disease?

- Concentrate on doing well on the exam and disregard any negative test-taking experiences in the past. Some people always do well on standardized tests; others have to develop this skill though practice and experience. If you have struggled with standardized tests, try to block out any previous negative experiences. Remember, you have spent years preparing for this exam, and the PANRE is designed to test your accumulated knowledge and skills as a physician assistant using a test that is fair, reasonable, and consistent.

CHAPTER 11

Organ System List (Overview)

ORGAN SYSTEMS TESTED ON THE PANRE

1. Cardiovascular

Circulatory system: Transports nutrients and gases to cells and tissues throughout the body.

Lymphatic system: A system of vessels containing lymph, which is a fluid that contains lymphocytes for assissting with immune response. The system also helps to drain interstitial fluid and transport dietary fats, inculding lipids and fat-soluble vitamins.

2. Dermatologic

Integumentary system: Protects the internal structures of the body from damage, prevents dehydration, stores fat, and produces vitamins and hormones.

3. EENT (Ears, Eyes, Nose, and Throat)

Sensory organs: Ears (hearing), eyes (sight), and nose (smell); Internal passage: Throat (food intake, air intake, and expulsion).

4. Endocrine

Endocrine system: Helps to maintain growth and homeostasis within the body through glands that excrete hormones into tissue and blood in the body.

5. Gastrointestinal/Nutritional

Digestive system: Breaks down food polymers into smaller molecules to provide energy and cellular building blocks for the body.

6. Genitourinary

Urinary/Excretory systems: Remove wastes and maintain water balance in the body.

7. Hematologic

Circulatory system: Transports nutrients and gases to cells and tissues throughout the body.

8. Infectious Diseases

Infectious disease: The presence of a microscopic pathological organism that has infected the host, such as bacteria, parasites, viruses, or fungi.

9. Musculoskeletal

Muscular system: Enables movement of the body.

Skeletal system: Supports and protects the body while giving it shape and form.

10. Neurologic System

Nervous system: Monitors and coordinates internal organ function and responds to changes in the external environment.

11. Psychiatry/Behavioral

Psychiatry/ Behavioral: These mental disorders include various affective, behavioral, cognitive, and perceptual abnormalities.

12. Pulmonary

Respiratory system: Provides the body with oxygen via gas exchange between air from the outside environment and gases in the blood.

13. Reproductive

Reproductive system: Enables the production of offspring through sexual reproduction.

PART IV

PRACTICE TEST

CHAPTER 12

Practice Test

Directions: Choose the option that best answers the question.

1. Which of the following medications is commonly administered for the prevention of deep venous thromboses?
   (A) Aspirin
   (B) Prednisone
   (C) IV immunoglobulin
   (D) Heparin
   (E) Danazol

2. A 15-month-old boy presents to the pediatrician with his mother. The boy's history is significant only for a delivery via C-section at 36 weeks after signs of fetal distress during labor. The mother is concerned that her child is not developing normally. He has not met developmental milestones of sitting, rolling, or crawling. Which of the following is the most accurate diagnosis?
   (A) Bell's palsy
   (B) Cerebral palsy
   (C) Erb's palsy
   (D) Down syndrome
   (E) Sarcoidosis

3. A 12-year-old female presents to her PCP with her mother who states that the child has had frequent bouts of "bronchitis" this winter. She also notes that she has occasionally had trouble with wheezing when running laps with her soccer team. She states that this happens 2 to 3 times/week. She states that it does not really affect her activity too much. Examination reveals normal breath sounds. Pulmonary function testing shows decreased FEV1, which reverses after a bronchodilator. What is the most likely diagnosis?
   (A) Hyperventilation syndrome
   (B) Mild intermittent asthma
   (C) Mild persistent asthma
   (D) Bronchiolitis
   (E) None of the above

4. A patient being treated with chlorothiazide to control hypertension may require supplementation with which of the following?
   (A) Selenium
   (B) Potassium
   (C) Lithium
   (D) Zinc
   (E) Iron

5. Which of the following is appropriate for maintenance treatment of pernicious anemia?
   (A) Ferrous sulfate
   (B) Vitamin B_{12}
   (C) Vitamin D
   (D) Erythropoeitin
   (E) Folic acid

6. A 72-year-old male presents to his PCP complaining of dyspnea and fatigue. Examination reveals an opening snap and a rumbling diastolic murmur heard loudest at the apex. What is the most likely diagnosis?
   (A) Mitral stenosis due to congenital heart disease
   (B) Mitral regurgitation due to rheumatic heart disease
   (C) Aortic stenosis due to congenital heart disease
   (D) Mitral stenosis due to rheumatic heart disease
   (E) Aortic regurgitation due to rheumatic heart disease

7. A 36-year-old woman presents with myalgias, arthralgias, nausea, vomiting, and hypotension. Adrenocorticotropic hormone (ACTH) stimulation test shows an elevation of cortisol level of 11μg (baseline is 9μg/dl). Which of the following is the most appropriate diagnosis?
   (A) Hypokalemia
   (B) Fibromyalgia
   (C) Addison's disease
   (D) Cushing's disease
   (E) Rheumatoid arthritis

8. Which of the following refers to mild contractions that occur after the sixth week of pregnancy but do not signal the start of labor?
   (A) P-5 contractions
   (B) Lamaze contractions
   (C) Braxton Hicks contractions
   (D) GDT contractions
   (E) Chadwick's contractions

9. Which of the following is appropriate treatment for individuals with acute coronary syndrome?
   (A) Morphine
   (B) Oxygen
   (C) Nitroglycerine
   (D) Aspirin
   (E) All of the above

10. A 24-year-old female presents with a severe headache, very high fever, and nuchal rigidity. She is exhibiting Brudzinski's and Babinski's signs. Which one of the following procedures would you have to perform before doing a spinal tap on this patient?
    (A) Blood culture
    (B) Check tendon stretch reflexes
    (C) Urinalysis
    (D) Ophthalmoscopy
    (E) Swab of nasopharynx

11. A 21-year-old female who was recently treated by her PCP for a vaginal infection has been out celebrating her birthday and presents to the emergency room with her friends. She complains of tachycardia, flushing, headache, shortness of breath, nausea, vomiting, and confusion. She states that she only had two drinks, and her friends confirm the history. What medication is she using to treat her "vaginal infection?"
    (A) Omeprazole (Prilosec)
    (B) Pyridoxine (Nestrex)
    (C) Norepinephrine (Levophed)
    (D) Metronidazole (Flagyl)
    (E) Penicillin VK (Pen VK)

12. Which of the following medications is used to treat urinary incontinence?
    (A) Tolterodine
    (B) Fluoroquinolone
    (C) Doxycycline
    (D) Vasodilators
    (E) Calcium channel blockers

13. Which of the following is the drug of choice for the treatment of diarrhea caused by *Cyclospora* infection?
    (A) TMP/SMX
    (B) Sulfadiazine
    (C) Sulfisoxazole
    (D) Cefepime
    (E) Metronidazole

14. A 65-year-old male presents to his PCP complaining of epigastric pain, weight loss, and jaundice. He has a 40 packs/year history of smoking. Examination reveals hepatomegaly and generalized abdominal tenderness. Laboratory reveals alkaline phosphatase of 550 U/L and a total bilirubin of 15 mg/dL. What is the most likely diagnosis?
    (A) Peptic ulcer disease
    (B) Cholecystitis
    (C) Pancreatic cancer
    (D) Ulcerative colitis
    (E) Gastric cancer

15. A 22-year-old male with a history of intravenous drug use presents with pleuritic chest pain, difficulty breathing, cough, and a fever of 102.4°F. Which of the following are the most appropriate diagnosis and etiologic agent?
    (A) Pericarditis/Influenza
    (B) Endocarditis/Staph aureus
    (C) Myocarditis/Coxsackie virus
    (D) Endocarditis/Strep viridans
    (E) Myocarditis/Toxoplasma

16. A 60-year-old male presents to his PCP with his son. The patient has been drinking heavily and skipping meals. His drinking has gradually worsened after losing his job and divorcing his wife. He is experiencing weakness, emotional lability, and myalgias. Examination reveals gait disturbance, 2/5 reflexes in all extremities, and ptosis. The patient is deficient in which of the following vitamins?
    (A) Niacin (Vitamin B_3)
    (B) Thiamine (Vitamin B_1)
    (C) Cobalamin (Vitamin B_{12})
    (D) Riboflavin (Vitamin B_2)
    (E) Pyridoxine (Vitamin B_6)

17. Which of the following refers to a buildup of collagen in the skin?
    (A) Polymyositis
    (B) Heberden's nodes
    (C) Reiter syndrome
    (D) Contact dermatitis
    (E) Scleroderma

18. Infection by which of the following is considered a risk factor for Hodgkin's lymphoma?
    (A) *Cryptococcus neoformans*
    (B) *Blastocystis hominis*
    (C) *Helicobacter pylori*
    (D) *Adenovirus*
    (E) *Epstein-Barr virus*

19. Which of the following medications is an abortifacient?
    (A) Misoprostol
    (B) Albuterol
    (C) Metformin
    (D) Corticotropin
    (E) Meloxicam

20. A 35-year-old female of Middle Eastern descent presents to her gynecologist with complaints of genital ulcers. She has also had oral ulcers, decreased visual acuity, and arthralgias. She denies any extramarital affairs and her husband has been asymptomatic. Examination reveals oral stomatitis and ulcers on the external genitalia. What is the most likely diagnosis?
    (A) Genital herpes
    (B) Syphilis
    (C) Stevens-Johnson syndrome
    (D) Behçet syndrome
    (E) Viral exanthema

21. Which of the following refers to a glandular disorder that characteristically manifests as dry mouth and dry eyes?
    (A) Tay-Sachs disease
    (B) Mononucleosis
    (C) Reiter syndrome
    (D) Raynaud's phenomenon
    (E) Sjögren's syndrome

22. Which of the following is a useful tool to confirm the diagnosis of dermatitis that develops on skin exposed to the sun?
    (A) KOH prep
    (B) Acetowhitening
    (C) Erythrocyte sedimentation rate
    (D) Photopatch test
    (E) Gram stain

23. A 27-year-old female with a history of Grave's disease, taking small dosages of propylthiouracil, is in the 18th week of pregnancy. She presents with a diffuse goiter and heavy thyrotoxicosis. Which of the following is the proper treatment for this patient?
(A) Thyroidectomy
(B) Beta-blockers
(C) Radioiodine therapy
(D) Methotrexate (Trexate)
(E) Increase dosage of propylthiouracil

24. Which of the following is a cyanotic type of congenital heart defect?
(A) Patent ductus arteriosus
(B) Atrioventricular septal defect
(C) Atrial septal defect
(D) Truncus arteriosus
(E) Ventricular septal defect

25. A 28-year-old Iraq War veteran presents to his PCP complaining of insomnia. Further questioning reveals that he has disturbing dreams and memories of specific events during the war. He has been drinking heavily in order to relieve these symptoms and to help him sleep. He will often have outbursts of anger toward his wife and children over very minor events. Prior to his deployment, he enjoyed training for marathons, but he has little interest in running now. He states that when he is out for a run, he will become overwhelmed with the fear that there are roadside bombs planted in his suburban neighborhood. What is the most likely diagnosis?
(A) Major depression
(B) Generalized anxiety disorder
(C) Post-traumatic stress disorder
(D) Alcoholism
(E) Bipolar disorder

26. Individuals who suffer from chronic kidney disease should avoid a diet rich in which of the following?
(A) Protein
(B) Green vegetables
(C) Wheat
(D) Corn
(E) Nightshade vegetables

27. A 70-year-old female with diabetes and CHF presents to her PCP complaining of fatigue and a "racing heart beat." Examination reveals BP 150/80. Pulse is irregularly irregular at 170 bpm. Cardiac exam reveals tachycardia and an irregularly irregular rhythm. EKG shows tachycardia, left axis deviation, and a wavy baseline with no defined P wave. Which of the following is the most likely diagnosis?
(A) CHF exacerbation
(B) DKA
(C) Atrial fibrillation
(D) Ventricular fibrillation
(E) Myocardial infarction

28. A 60-year-old woman presents to her PCP with a complaint of severe pain on the left side of the face, mostly located around the cheek. The patient states that even a very light touch can provoke excruciating pain. On exam, she weighs 135 pounds, which is 10 pounds lower than her baseline. On palpation of the left side of the face, no lesions are noted, but pain is present out of proportion with physical exam. Which of the following is the most likely diagnosis?
(A) Trigeminal neuralgia
(B) Migraine headache
(C) Multiple sclerosis
(D) Post-herpetic neuralgia
(E) Hemi-facial spasm

29. A 35-year-old female presents with an uncomplicated urinary tract infection. What is the most likely etiologic agent?
(A) *Bacillus cereus*
(B) *Escherichia coli*
(C) *Balantidium coli*
(D) *Absidia corymbifera*
(E) *Citrobacter diversus*

30. An 80-year-old female presents to her PCP complaining of chest discomfort and shortness of breath. Her daughter brought her in because she fainted at a family reunion. Examination reveals a IV/VI systolic crescendo-decrescendo murmur heard loudest at the right sternal border. What is the most likely diagnosis?
(A) Aortic stenosis
(B) Mitral valve prolapse
(C) Aortic regurgitation
(D) Vasovagal syncope
(E) Myocardial infarction

31. Which of the following is the proper first line of treatment for individuals with diverticulitis?
(A) High-fiber diet
(B) Proton pump inhibitors (PPIs)
(C) Gastroprokinetic agent
(D) Antibiotics
(E) NSAIDs

32. A 55-year-old obese male presents to his PCP with complaints of persistent fatigue. Recently, he has started falling asleep at traffic lights. He states that he never can get enough rest and that he is tired even upon awakening. He often has a headache in the morning. His wife has moved to another bedroom because of his loud snoring. What is the most likely diagnosis?
(A) Depression
(B) Sleep apnea
(C) Fibromyalgia
(D) Sleep disorder
(E) Sinusitis

33. Megaloblastic anemia is typically caused by deficiency of which of the following?
(A) Vitamin C
(B) Vitamin B_{12}
(C) Vitamin B_6
(D) Vitamin K
(E) Vitamin E

34. Hordeola are typically caused by which of the following?
(A) *Candida albicans*
(B) *Streptococcus pneumoniae*
(C) *Haemophilus influenza*
(D) *Streptococcus agalactiae*
(E) *Staphylococcus aureus*

35. A 7-year-old female with a history of seasonal allergies presents to her PCP with her mother complaining of cracking, dry, and peeling hands. Her mother reports that the condition started when the patient began to play hockey last year. Topical steroids clear the condition, but it always returns. What is the most likely diagnosis?
(A) Psoriasis
(B) Tinea corporis
(C) Seborrheic dermatitis
(D) Atopic dermatitis
(E) Dermatitis herpetiformis

36. Levothyroxine is commonly used to treat which of the following disorders?
(A) Hyperparathyroidism
(B) Thyrotoxicosis
(C) Hypothyroidism
(D) Hypoparathyroidism
(E) Grave's disease

37. Which of the following medications is commonly administered for the prevention of tuberculosis?
(A) Aminophylline
(B) Amiodarone
(C) Valproic acid
(D) Ketoconazole
(E) Isoniazid

38. Which of the following modalities is used to differentiate gram-negative from gram-positive bacteria?
(A) Darkfield microscopy
(B) Sputum culture
(C) Western blot
(D) Giemsa stain
(E) Gram stain

39. An 18-year-old female G1P0 is 37 weeks pregnant. She presents to the emergency department complaining of headache and edema in hands and feet. Examination reveals BP of 150/80. Urinalysis reveals 2+ protein. What is the most likely diagnosis?
(A) Urinary tract infection
(B) Pre-eclampsia
(C) Essential hypertension
(D) Nephrotic syndrome
(E) Eclampsia

40. Infection by *Bacillus anthracis* is most effectively treated by which of the following medications?
(A) Ciprofloxacin
(B) Clarithromycin
(C) TMP/SMX
(D) Ceftriaxone
(E) Cefepime

41. Which of the following is a seizure medication commonly prescribed for the treatment of petit mal seizures?
(A) Clonazepam
(B) Felbamate
(C) Gabapentin
(D) Phenytoin
(E) Valproic acid

42. Which of the following disorders is likely to be characterized by episodic vertigo, tinnitus, ear pressure, and hearing impairment?
(A) Achondrogenesis
(B) Ménière's disease
(C) Munchausen syndrome
(D) Legionnaire's disease
(E) Epistaxis

43. A 12-year-old male with a history of asthma presents to his PCP with complaints of sinus congestion, runny nose, and facial pain. Physical examination reveals a mostly occluded nasal cavity on the right side because of obstruction by large grapelike masses. What would be an expected finding under the patient's allergy list?
(A) Amoxicillin
(B) Cephalexin
(C) Levofloxacin
(D) ASA (acetylsalicylic acid; aspirin)
(E) Naproxen

44. A 40-year-old female presents to her PCP complaining of fatigue, malaise, dizziness and "dark spots" on the hands and lips. Examination reveals BP 100/60. Laboratories reveal low sodium and elevated potassium. What is the most likely diagnosis?
(A) Anorexia nervosa
(B) Diabetes type II
(C) Hyperaldosteronism
(D) Addison's disease
(E) Melasma

45. Which of the following is the preferred current medication of choice for the treatment of gonorrhea?
(A) Norfloxacin
(B) Ofloxacin
(C) Levofloxacin
(D) Ceftriaxone
(E) Ciprofloxacin

46. Which of the following may exacerbate heart failure by reducing oxygen flow to the heart?
(A) Arrhythmia
(B) Hypertension
(C) Myocardial injury
(D) Anemia
(E) Sleep apnea

47. A 45-year-old female presents to her PCP with painful swelling under the right mandible that started suddenly. The pain is worse with eating and is associated with fever and decreased saliva. Examination reveals tender submandibular swelling and purulent discharge from the submandibular salivary gland. What is the most likely diagnosis?
(A) Mumps
(B) Lymphoma
(C) Siladenitis
(D) Cat-scratch disease
(E) Ludwig's angina

48. A 35-year-old male presents to his PCP with the complaint of vertigo, hearing loss, and high-pitched tinnitus. Examination of the head and neck is normal; however, referral for audiogram reveals severe hearing loss in the right ear with a normal audiogram on the left. What is the most likely diagnosis?
(A) Acoustic neuroma
(B) Benign paroxysmal positional vertigo (BPPV)
(C) Ménière's disease
(D) Sudden sensorineural hearing loss
(E) None of the above

49. Which of the following medications may be used to suppress cortisol production in patients with Cushing's syndrome?
(A) Ketoconazole
(B) Prednisone
(C) Fludrocortisone acetate
(D) Clotrimazole
(E) Dexamethazone

50. A 65-year-old male presents to his PCP with paresthesias, fatigue, mood swings, and inability to focus. A CBC shows an increased MCV, and a smear reveals megaloblasts. He has been reading about his symptoms on the Internet and thinks he might have pernicious anemia. Examination reveals palor, decreased vibratory and position sense, and decreased reflexes throughout all extremities. Which of the following vitamin deficiencies is the patient suffering from?
    (A) Riboflavin (Vitamin B₂)
    (B) Ascorbic acid (Vitamin C)
    (C) Retinoic acid (Vitamin A)
    (D) Cobalamin (Vitamin B₁₂)
    (E) Phylloquinone (Vitamin K)

51. Which of the following is a loop diuretic used in the treatment of chronic hypertension?
    (A) Furosemide
    (B) Mannitol
    (C) Triamterine
    (D) Chlorothiazide
    (E) Amiloride

52. Analysis of a stool sample is helpful to accurately confirm the diagnosis of which of the following?
    (A) Barrett's esophagus
    (B) Meningitis
    (C) Strongyloidiasis
    (D) Otitis Media
    (E) Necrotizing fasciitis

53. A 19-year-old female presents to the emergency room with severe headache, fever, and vomiting, which her mother reports started suddenly "like the flu." Examination reveals drowsiness and confusion. An electroencephalograph (EEG) shows sharp waves in both of the temporal lobes. Cerebrospinal fluid (CSF) reveals elevated protein and white blood cells with normal glucose. The patient is diagnosed with encephalitis. Which of the following is the most likely organism causing her condition?
    (A) Herpes simplex virus type 1 (HSV-1)
    (B) *Staphylococcus aureus*
    (C) *Listeria monocytogenes*
    (D) *Streptococcus pneumoniae*
    (E) Coxsackie virus

54. Pleural mesothelioma is a pulmonary disorder most commonly caused by exposure to which of the following?
    (A) Asbestos
    (B) Nicotine
    (C) Dust
    (D) Carbon monoxide
    (E) Fiberglass

55. A 28-year-old female with a history of pelvic inflammatory disease presents to her PCP with a history of irregular periods. She states that her period was one week late and then started one week ago and has not stopped. She also complains of pelvic pain and dizziness. Examination reveals a right adnexal mass. What is the most likely diagnosis?
    (A) Appendicitis
    (B) Ectopic pregnancy
    (C) Ruptured ovarian cyst
    (D) Pelvic inflammatory disease
    (E) Irritable bowel syndrome

56. Which of the following is the standard treatment for chronic myelocytic leukemia (CML)?
    (A) Nicardipine
    (B) Carbamazepine
    (C) Warfarin
    (D) Amlodipine
    (E) Imatinib

57. A 16-year-old male presents to his PCP complaining of a mildly pruritic rash that started two days ago. About a week before the rash, he had a large "patch" on his trunk, which resolved. Past medical history is non-contributory. He is not sexually active, and family history is essentially negative. Physical examination reveals salmon-colored plaques with light scale that are oriented in a "Christmas tree" pattern. KOH prep is negative. What is the most likely diagnosis?
    (A) Secondary syphilis
    (B) Viral exanthem
    (C) Psoriasis
    (D) Pityriasis rosea
    (E) Tinea corporis

58. A 25-year-old female who is 36 weeks pregnant presents to the emergency room with vaginal bleeding. Her husband reports that she suddenly started with severe persistent abdominal pain and severe bleeding 20 minutes before presenting to the emergency room. Her prenatal care has been inconsistent, but during most of her visits she has been hypertensive. What is the most likely diagnosis?

(A) Placentia previa
(B) Pre-term labor
(C) Placental abruption
(D) Appendicitis
(E) Peptic ulcer disease

59. A 55-year-old female presents to her PCP with the complaint of joint stiffness and pain. The stiffness is worse in the morning and lasts for more than an hour after waking. She also complains of fatigue and depression that has worsened over the past six months. Examination reveals swelling, erythema, and warmth in the elbows and knees bilaterally. Laboratory examination reveals an elevated ESR and positive Rheumatoid factor. What is the most likely diagnosis?

(A) Fibromyalgia
(B) Rheumatoid arthritis
(C) Lupus
(D) Lyme disease
(E) Osteoarthritis

60. A 43-year-old female with two healthy children is diagnosed with a complete hydatidiform mole (gestational trophoblastic disease). Which of the following procedures is required to treat this condition?

(A) Chemotherapy
(B) Radiation
(C) Dilation and curettage
(D) Mifepristone (Mifeprex)
(E) Hysterectomy

61. Which of the following is the predominant bacterial pathogen responsible for chronic gastritis?

(A) *Clostridium septicum*
(B) *Brucella melitensis*
(C) *Bacillus cereus*
(D) *Helicobacter pylori*
(E) *Enterobacteriaceae*

62. A 16-year-old Hispanic male presents with his mother for a well check. Family history is significant for diabetes on both sides of the family. Examination reveals a well-developed obese male with a velvety hyper-pigmented appearance to the neck and axilla. What is the diagnosis and the most important screening measure to be taken at this patient's visit?

(A) Tinea corporis, KOH prep
(B) Acanthosis nigricans, blood glucose
(C) Acanthosis nigricans, dermatology referral
(D) Hidradenitis superativa, oral antibiotics
(E) Tinea corporis, nutrition counseling

63. A 25-year-old female presents for a well check. Examination reveals a holosystolic murmur at the apex radiating to the axilla with an associated click. Which of the following would be the most appropriate diagnosis?

(A) Mitral valve prolapse
(B) Aortic stenosis
(C) Mitral stenosis
(D) Hypertrophic cardiomyopathy
(E) Tricuspid stenosis

64. A 12-year-old boy is brought into the emergency room by his mother. She states that he has been convulsing for the last 45 minutes. The boy has a history of epilepsy, and his treatment was modified two weeks ago. The patient is in a generalized tonic clonic seizure upon presentation to the ER. Which of the following medications is the most appropriate for this situation?

(A) Valproic acid
(B) Valium (diazepam)
(C) Carbamazepine
(D) Gabapentin
(E) Ethosuximide

65. Which of the following is the major side effect of angiotensin-converting enzyme (ACE) inhibitors?

(A) Neuropathy
(B) Vomiting
(C) Nausea
(D) Dry cough
(E) Wheezing

66. A 25-year-old Caucasian female presents to her PCP with complaints of abdominal pain, weight loss, fatigue, and chronic diarrhea. Examination reveals a thin, cooperative female in no acute distress. She is pale and has generalized abdominal tenderness without rebound or guarding. Laboratories reveal HgB of 9.5 g/dl, MCV 68, and an elevated ESR. What is the most likely diagnosis?
    (A) Laxative abuse
    (B) Peptic ulcer disease
    (C) Crohn's disease
    (D) Ischemic colitis
    (E) Pancreatic cancer

67. A 17-year-old female presents to the emergency room complaining of pelvic pain associated with vaginal discharge. She became sexually active for the first time 2 months ago. Examination reveals cervicitis with a thick yellow discharge. Bimanual exam reveals cervical motion tenderness. Laboratory examination reveals a quantitative Beta hCG and a WBC of 12,000. What is the most likely diagnosis?
    (A) Pelvic inflammatory disease
    (B) Ectopic pregnancy
    (C) Ruptured ovarian cyst
    (D) Endometriosis
    (E) Bacterial vaginosis

68. Which of the following medications is commonly used in conjunction with peginterferon for treatment of chronic hepatitis C?
    (A) Interferon beta-1b
    (B) Abacavir
    (C) Ribavirin
    (D) Didanosine
    (E) Emtricitabine

69. Which of the following is the most common etiology of acromegaly?
    (A) *Campylobacter jejuni*
    (B) Adrenocortical carcinoma
    (C) Adenovirus
    (D) *Bacteroides fragilis*
    (E) Benign pituitary tumor

70. A 55-year-old male with DM presents to the emergency room with a complaint of malaise, shortness of breath, nausea, and "indigestion." He states that he has had nausea and "cold sweats" when walking for the past several months. Examination reveals BP 80/50 and a pulse of 50. EKG reveals ST elevation in leads II, III, and aVF. What is the most likely diagnosis?
    (A) Symptomatic bradycardia
    (B) Hypovolemic shock
    (C) Inferior myocardial infarction
    (D) Atrial fibrillation
    (E) Anterior myocardial infarction

71. Which of the following medications used to treat attention deficit hyperactivity disorder (ADHD) is a non-stimulant drug?
    (A) Atomoxetine
    (B) Buproprion
    (C) Levoamphetamine
    (D) Lisdexamfetamine dimesylate
    (E) Methylphenidate

72. A cardiac patient who experiences discomfort upon performing any physical activity is most likely experiencing which of the following functional classes of heart disease?
    (A) I
    (B) II
    (C) III
    (D) IV
    (E) V

73. Consumption of which of the following vitamins is effective for preventing rickets?
    (A) Vitamin A
    (B) Vitamin D
    (C) Vitamin K
    (D) Vitamin E
    (E) Vitamin C

74. A 45-year-old woman presents to the emergency room with her husband. She complains of a severe headache of sudden onset, which she describes as "the worst headache of my life." The patient has no history of trauma. Physical exam reveals somnolence, nuchal rigidity, and a BP of 170/105. What is the most likely etiology of this patient's condition?
    (A) Subarachnoid hemorrhage
    (B) Tumor
    (C) Metabolic disease
    (D) Central nervous system (CNS) infection
    (E) Trauma

75. A 25-year-old female patient presents at the clinic with sharp RUQ pain, nausea, and vomiting. A complete CBC, AST/ALT along with an Amylase and Lipase has been ordered. What imaging test should be done to rule out Cholelithiasis?
    (A) Hydroxy iminodiaetic acid scan (HIDA)
    (B) Computer tomography (CT)
    (C) Gallbladder ultrasound
    (D) X-ray series of abdomen
    (E) Endoscopic retrograde cholangio-pancrea-tography (ERCP)

76. Lyme disease is a spirochetal infection caused by which of the following bacteria?
    (A) *Listeria monocytogenes*
    (B) *Nocardia asteroides*
    (C) *Rickettsia rickettsii*
    (D) *Borrelia burgdorferi*
    (E) *Neisseria meningitides*

77. A 30-year-old male presents with complaints of irritability, hyperpigmentation, decreased appetite, and weight loss. Physical examination reveals 3/5 strength in all extremities and hypotension. Which of the following is the most appropriate diagnosis?
    (A) Grave's disease
    (B) Cushing's disease
    (C) Addison's disease
    (D) Wilson's disease
    (E) Diabetes mellitus

78. A 50-year-old female presents to the emergency room after falling from her bicycle. During the crash, she put out her right hand to catch herself. Examination reveals tenderness over the base of the thumb in the "anatomical snuffbox." What is the most likely diagnosis?
    (A) Fracture of the first metacarpal
    (B) Fracture of the scaphoid
    (C) Fracture of the distal radius
    (D) Tendonitis
    (E) Fracture of the distal ulna

79. A 55-year-old female being treated for stage IV ductal carcinoma presents with polyuria and poly-dipsia. Urinalysis reveals an osmolality of <250 mOsm/kg, and serum osmolality is high. Patient is given ADH and has a positive response. Which of the following is the most likely diagnosis?
    (A) Diabetes mellitus type II
    (B) Diabetes insipidus
    (C) Urinary tract infection
    (D) Addison's disease
    (E) Impaired renal function

80. A 35-year-old female patient with a strong family history of headaches presents to the emergency room with a chief complaint of headache. She describes the pain as unilateral, 8/10 intensity, with associated photo- and phonophobia. She has been having these headaches since she was 13. Her mother had similar headaches that resolved somewhat after menopause. These symptoms keep the patient from performing her daily activities. Which of the following is the most likely diagnosis?
    (A) Migraine
    (B) Cluster headaches
    (C) Intracranial hemorrhage
    (D) Viral meningitis
    (E) Cerebral aneurysm

81. Which of the following is typically prescribed for maintenance treatment of chronic obstructive pulmonary disorder (COPD)?
    (A) Roflumilast
    (B) Fentanyl
    (C) Colcyrs
    (D) Clindamycin
    (E) Phentolamine

82. A 45-year-old high school teacher is brought to the emergency room by paramedics. She states that she was standing for 2 hours at a parade. She states that she felt "woozy," and bystanders report that she lost consciousness and fell to the ground. She was unconscious for only 2 or 3 minutes and had no confusion upon recovery. The paramedics report that the bystanders denied any seizure-like activity on the part of the patient. There is no history of prior episodes or any other medical problems. The physical examination is normal. What is the next step in the evaluation of the patient?
    (A) Cerebral MRI
    (B) Echocardiogram (Echo)
    (C) Electroencephalogram (EEG)
    (D) Electrocardiogram (EKG)
    (E) Complete blood count (CBC)

83. Deficiency of which of the following is the main etiology for beriberi?
    (A) Vitamin A
    (B) Biotin
    (C) Riboflavin
    (D) Folate
    (E) Thiamine

84. A 60-year-old male presents to his PCP for a routine physical. Current medications include Atenolol 50 mg and HCTZ 12.5 mg. He has a 40 packs/year history of smoking. Examination reveals a pulsatile mass in the epigastrium. What is the most likely diagnosis?
    (A) Peptic ulcer disease
    (B) Umbilical hernia
    (C) Abdominal aortic aneurysm
    (D) Cholecystitis
    (E) None of the above

85. Which of the following should be administered to prevent atherothrombosis in patients with diabetes mellitus type 2?
    (A) Vitamin C
    (B) Glyburide
    (C) Repaglinide
    (D) Metformin
    (E) Aspirin

86. An 8-year-old boy presents with his mother to his pediatrician. She is worried about his performance at school. The boy's teacher reports that the boy often stares into space for a few seconds and then asks questions about the subjects that were just covered. The patient sometimes blinks excessively during these episodes and does not respond to the teacher. What would be the most appropriate medication for this diagnosis?
    (A) Phenytoin
    (B) Carbamazepine
    (C) Diazepam
    (D) Phenobarbital
    (E) Ethosuximide

87. Which of the following medications administered for the treatment of depression has an effect on the action of both serotonin and norepinephrine?
    (A) Duloxetine (Cymbalta)
    (B) Sertraline (Zoloft)
    (C) Fluoxetine (Prozac)
    (D) Paroxetine (Paxil)
    (E) Citalopram (Celexa)

88. Which of the following is the primary drug class of choice for treatment of chronic angina?
    (A) Diuretics
    (B) Alpha-blockers
    (C) ACE inhibitors
    (D) Calcium channel blockers
    (E) Beta-blockers

89. Which can decrease the effectiveness of Warfarin (Coumadin)?
    (A) Vitamin D
    (B) Calcium
    (C) Selenium
    (D) Vitamin K
    (E) Zinc

90. A 51-year-old female presents with chorea, dystonia, and impaired gait. In addition, she has been exhibiting anxiety and a slowed thought process. Which of the following is the most appropriate diagnosis?
    (A) Huntington's disease
    (B) Multiple sclerosis
    (C) Parkinson's disease
    (D) Myasthenia gravis
    (E) Alzheimer's disease

91. A 3-year-old boy presents with his mother, who states that the child has been sleeping poorly, pulling at his ear, and complaining of pain in the right ear. She also states that he has been getting over a cold for the past week. Physical examination reveals a fever of 102°F and a bulging tympanic membrane. Based on the patient's history and physical examination, which of the following is the most appropriate diagnosis?
    (A) Acoustic neuroma
    (B) Ménière's disease
    (C) Ceruminosis
    (D) Otitis media
    (E) Labyrinthitis

92. A 75-year-old female patient presents with epigastric pain radiating to the back, jaundice, and weight loss. You have ordered a complete metabolic panel (CMP), amylase, trypsinogen test, and an endoscopic ultrasound (EUS). What is the suspected diagnosis?
    (A) Colon cancer
    (B) Stomach cancer
    (C) Liver cancer
    (D) Pancreatic cancer
    (E) Gall bladder cancer

93. A 23-year-old man is brought to the emergency room by paramedics after a bar fight. During the fight, he was hit in the head with a baseball bat. He presents with anisocoria and is rated at a 7 on the Glasgow coma scale. The CT scan shows a hyper-dense convex image between the brain and the skull. Which of the following interventions is the most appropriate for this patient's condition?
    (A) Anticoagulant therapy
    (B) Observation
    (C) Surgery
    (D) Antibiotic therapy
    (E) Sedation

94. A 65-year-old female presents to his PCP with her daughter who states that she has been depressed and with an atypical affect. She also has been complaining of pain in the arms and legs, constipation, and polydipsia. She was in good health when she started developing kidney stones and has frequently been in the ER. Examination reveals an apathetic affect, BP 150/80, and 4/5 strength in all extremities. Laboratories reveal a calcium of 11.0 mg/dl. What is the most likely diagnosis?
    (A) Osteoporosis
    (B) Hypothyroidism
    (C) Hyperparathyroidism
    (D) Essential hypertension
    (E) Renal artery stenosis

95. Administration of levonorgestrel/ethinyl estradiol can prevent the occurrence of which of the following?
    (A) Goiter
    (B) Gout
    (C) Pregnancy
    (D) Empyema
    (E) Diarrhea

96. Which of the following refers to spasms of the blood vessels in the fingers and toes?
    (A) Raynaud's phenomenon
    (B) Still's disease
    (C) Reiter syndrome
    (D) Dermatomytosis
    (E) Scheie syndrome

97. A 68-year-old female presents with primary hyperparathyroidism. She has parathyroid-related osteoporosis, and she has been found to have ectopic calcifications. Which of the following is the proper intervention to treat this condition?
    (A) Alendronate (Fosamax)
    (B) Parathyroidectomy
    (C) Calcium and vitamin D supplements
    (D) Radioiodine therapy
    (E) Levothyroxine (Synthroid)

98. A 19-year-old college student presents to the emergency room with a complaint of fever and neck stiffness. Brudzinski's sign is positive. Meningitis is suspected. Before a lumbar puncture can be ordered, the patient becomes somnolent and is not able to answer any questions coherently. What is the most important FIRST test to be ordered for this patient?
    (A) CT scan of the brain
    (B) Blood culture
    (C) Lumbar puncture
    (D) Electroencephalography (EEG)
    (E) Transcranial Doppler study

99. Which of the following is commonly prescribed for treatment of hypokalemia?
    (A) Oral calcium
    (B) IV magnesium
    (C) Oral phosphorus
    (D) Oral potassium
    (E) IV phosphorus

100. Each of the following pathogens is a common cause of bacterial conjunctivitis EXCEPT
    (A) *Staphylococcus aureus*
    (B) *Pseudomonas aeruginosa*
    (C) *Listeria monocytogenes*
    (D) *Streptococcus pneumoniae*
    (E) *Hemophilus influenzae*

101. Which of the following is the main etiology for genital herpes?
    (A) Herpes simplex virus type 1 (HSV-1)
    (B) Human immunodeficiency virus (HIV)
    (C) Candida albicans
    (D) Human papillomavirus (HPV)
    (E) Herpes simplex virus type 2 (HSV-2)

102. Which of the following medications is used for the treatment of nephrotic syndrome?
    (A) Naproxen
    (B) Meloxicam
    (C) Piroxicam
    (D) Ibuprofen
    (E) ACE inhibitors

103. Which of the following medications is commonly prescribed for maintenance treatment of Crohn's disease?
    (A) Prednisone
    (B) Mesalamine
    (C) Adefovir
    (D) Deferasirox
    (E) Tagamet

104. It is March, and a 7-year-old boy presents with his father to the emergency room complaining of sore throat, fever, and vomiting that started suddenly 5 hours ago. Examination reveals a fever of 102.7°F, 4+ tonsils with purulent exudate, beefy red uvula, and anterior cervical lymphadenopathy. What is the most common cause and appropriate treatment of the child's condition?
    (A) Viral, 5 days of azithromycin
    (B) Group A beta-hemolytic streptococci, 10 days of amoxicillin
    (C) Group A beta-hemolytic streptococci, 10 days of erythromycin
    (D) Epstein-Barr virus, supportive therapy
    (E) Adenovirus, supportive therapy

105. A 21-year-old male presents to his PCP with his mother because of recent odd behavior. She has noticed that he often neglects to bathe or brush his hair. He has recently lost his job because he was frequently hours late. When he did report to his job, he would often spend long periods of time appearing to be doing nothing. He has lost a great number of friends because of his odd behavior. His mother frequently misses phone calls because he has taken the phones off the hook due to worry that he is being "spied on." What is the most likely diagnosis?
    (A) Bipolar disorder
    (B) Obsessive compulsive disorder
    (C) Schizophrenia
    (D) Major depression
    (E) Borderline personality disorder

106. A 25-year-old Asian female in her first trimester of pregnancy presents with intermittent muscle weakness and fatigue. These episodes are brought on by exercise and resolve with rest, but with pregnancy they have been more persistent. She also states that she has periods of double vision and difficulty speaking and chewing. Which of the following medications is the most appropriate treatment?
    (A) Antibiotic therapy
    (B) Immunosuppressive therapy
    (C) Folic acid (B_9)
    (D) Cognitive behavioral psychotherapy
    (E) Ferrous sulfate (iron)

107. Cetirizine is commonly used to treat which of the following?
    (A) Tinnitus
    (B) Allergic rhinitis
    (C) Vertigo
    (D) Hypertension
    (E) Renal failure

108. An 18-month-old female presents with her mother, who states that the child has had a persistent cough since she was very young. The child did not present for her 12-month well check. However, since her 6-month check-up, she has fallen from the fiftieth percentile to the fifteenth percentile in height and weight. She has also been hospitalized recently for some sort of "stomach problem." Examination reveals a poorly developed child. Examination of the chest reveals coarse wheezes throughout. Sweat test is positive. What is the most likely diagnosis?
    (A) Cystic fibrosis
    (B) Asthma
    (C) Bronchiolitis
    (D) Pneumonia
    (E) GERD

109. A 21-year-old female presents to her PCP with her mother. Her mother has become concerned about her since her grades have been slipping at school. She had been away at school but moved home this year because of her failing grades. Further questioning revealed that her roommates "kicked her out" because her doll collection was taking over their apartment. She frequently misses class, because it takes her an hour to leave the house. She reports that she has to check the locks and the stove no less than 10 times. Her mother reports that she spends 2 hours in the bathroom in the morning and that the wallpaper is peeling off the walls due to her excessive showering. What is the most likely diagnosis?
    (A) Schizophrenia
    (B) Major depression
    (C) Bipolar disorder
    (D) Obsessive compulsive disorder
    (E) Histrionic personality disorder

110. Which of the following conditions refers to serum sodium levels of <136 mEq/L?
    (A) Hyphema
    (B) Hyponatremia
    (C) Hypospadias
    (D) Hypotonia
    (E) Hypokalemia

111. Which of the following medications may be prescribed for smoking cessation?
    (A) Carbamazepine
    (B) Bupropion
    (C) Haloperidol
    (D) Phenytoin
    (E) Clozapine

112. A 61-year-old Caucasian who is being treated for schizophrenia with thorazine presents with her caretaker, who complains that she is grimacing, sticking out her tongue, smacking her lips, and blinking frequently. Which of the following is the most likely diagnosis?
    (A) Alzheimers disease
    (B) Tardive dyskinesia
    (C) Neuroleptic malignant syndrome
    (D) Huntington's disease
    (E) Parkinson's disease

113. *Molluscum contagiosum* is a skin disorder caused by which of the following?
    (A) Parasite
    (B) Fungus
    (C) Virus
    (D) Bacteria
    (E) Allergy

114. A 35-year-old sales executive presents with his wife because she is concerned that he has given her an STD. Further questioning reveals that she is his fourth wife. They have been married for one year and for that year, he made her feel like a "queen." However, after a minor disappointment over the card he received for their anniversary, she has been concerned that he is having an affair. When you question the husband alone, he states that his wife clearly does not love him and that is why he has been involved with his secretary, who is "perfect." He has had five jobs in the past seven years. He reports that he will do really well with his sales numbers and then the "management will stop appreciating him," so he moves on to the next opportunity. What is the most likely diagnosis?
    (A) Narcissistic personality disorder
    (B) Obsessive compulsive disorder
    (C) Schizophrenia
    (D) Generalized anxiety disorder
    (E) Major depression

115. Body dysmorphic disorder can be effectively treated by which of the following?
    (A) SSRIs
    (B) MAIOs
    (C) Tricyclic antidepressants
    (D) Phenothiazines
    (E) SGAs

116. Meloxicam is commonly prescribed for treatment of which of the following disorders?
    (A) Acute kidney failure
    (B) Hypotension
    (C) Rheumatoid arthritis
    (D) Chronic kidney failure
    (E) Malaria

117. A 37-year-old female with a recent diagnosis of HTN presents to the emergency room with the complaint of palpitations, headache, and diaphoresis. Her symptoms have been episodic for the past two months. Current medications include Enalapril 40 mg once daily, Carvedilol 25 mg twice daily, and Amlodipine 10 mg. She states that she has been compliant with her medications but that her BP continues to "spike." There is no family history of hypertension. Examination reveals BP 180/110. Patient is diaphoretic, tremulous, and anxious. Cardiac exam reveals tachycardia. Which of the following is NOT an appropriate part of this patient's treatment plan?
    (A) 24-hour urine for catecholamines
    (B) Thyroid function tests
    (C) EKG
    (D) Continue to titrate BP medications
    (E) CT of abdomen

118. Metformin should not be administered to diabetic patients with which of the following disorders?
    (A) Chronic asthma
    (B) Crohn's disease
    (C) Kidney failure
    (D) Celiac disease
    (E) AIDS

119. A 40-year-old woman presents to her PCP with a chief complaint of moderate bilateral headache for five months. She started pursuing a new degree five months ago and has been spending a lot more time on the computer. She states that typing for long periods of time triggers her headaches. She states that ibuprofen usually helps to alleviate the headaches. The patient also reports that she saw her dentist seven months ago for nighttime teeth grinding. Physical exam reveals muscle spasm around the head and neck. Neurologic exam is normal. Which of the following interventions is required to diagnose this condition?
    (A) Urinalysis
    (B) History and physical examination
    (C) Cerebrospinal fluid (CSF)
    (D) Blood culture
    (E) Ultrasonography

120. A 70-year-old man is brought into the office by his wife. She believes his health is deteriorating and she wants to know what is wrong with him. The patient states that he has had a hard time writing checks lately because his writing is barely legible. He has also become "clumsy," falling twice in the last month. Examination reveals a "pill rolling" tremor of the right hand while at rest, as well as difficulty initiating movement when standing up from the chair. Which of the following is the most appropriate diagnosis?
(A) Parkinson's disease
(B) Huntington's disease
(C) Multiple sclerosis
(D) Lou Gehrig's disease
(E) Myasthenia gravis

121. A 65-year-old male presents to his PCP for a routine physical with complaints of fatigue, constipation, and mucus in the stool. Examination reveals heme positive stool but is otherwise negative. However, CBC reveals a HgB of 10.2 g/dl and an MCV of 68. What is the most important next test?
(A) CT scan abdomen and pelvis
(B) Colonoscopy
(C) Barium swallow
(D) Stool specimen for *Helobacter pylori*
(E) Abdominal ultrasound

122. Each of the following medications may be used to treat rheumatoid arthritis EXCEPT
(A) Methotrexate
(B) Rituximab
(C) Sulfasalazine
(D) Lovastatin
(E) Leflunomide

123. Dextromethorphan is commonly used in the treatment which of the following?
(A) Rheumatoid arthritis
(B) Mastitis
(C) Hypothyroidism
(D) Cough
(E) Hodgkin's lymphoma

124. Which of the following medications is commonly prescribed for maintenance treatment of genital herpes?
(A) Methotrexate
(B) Acyclovir
(C) Ciprofloxacin
(D) ASA
(E) Metronidazole

125. A 45-year-old musician presents to the emergency room with a complaint of tremors. He has had a mild tremor in both hands for three years, but the problem is worsening. It is starting to affect his performance on the piano, and he has even noticed a slight "vibrato" in his singing voice. He feels better if he has a couple of beers before he gets on stage. He is worried that he may share the same fate as his mother, who was a famous musician whose career was cut short by similar symptoms. Physical exam is essentially normal. What is the most appropriate line of treatment for this patient?
(A) Beta2-blockers (β_2)
(B) Benzodiazepines
(C) No medications
(D) Alcohol
(E) Antidepressants

126. A 48-year-old man presents with a vascular, tri-angular, elevated conjunctival mass encroaching on his cornea. Which of the following is the most appropriate diagnosis?
(A) Orbital cellulitis
(B) Blepharitis
(C) Chalazion
(D) Pinguccula
(E) Pterygium

127. A newborn boy is being evaluated for small head circumference and low birth weight of 4 lbs. The mother reports that she did not have prenatal care. Physical examination reveals a smooth philtrum, thin vermillion, and small palpebral fissures. Upon further questioning, the mother reports that she did drink heavily during the pregnancy. According to the patient's history and physical examination, which of the following would be the most appropriate diagnosis?
(A) Down syndrome
(B) Trisomy 8
(C) Williams syndrome
(D) Fetal alcohol syndrome (FAS)
(E) Meconium aspiration syndrome

128. Which of the following diagnostic procedures is used to identify the pathogen Treponema pallidum?
(A) India ink preparation
(B) Giemsa stain
(C) KOH preparation
(D) Gram stain
(E) Darkfield examination

129. Albuterol is commonly prescribed to treat which of the following?
    (A) Legionnaire's disease
    (B) Salmonellosis
    (C) Chronic lymphocytic leukemia
    (D) Erectile dysfunction
    (E) Asthma

130. An 80-year-old female presents to her PCP with a complaint of sore throat and painful tongue. Examination reveals a white coating on the tongue and soft palate that scrapes off easily, revealing erythema. What is the most likely diagnosis?
    (A) Oral candidiasis
    (B) Hairy leukoplakia
    (C) Herpes stomatitis
    (D) Glossitis
    (E) None of the above

131. A 25-year-old Caucasian female presents to her PCP with complaints of abdominal pain, weight loss, fatigue, and chronic diarrhea. Examination reveals a thin, cooperative female in no acute distress. She is pale and has generalized abdominal tenderness without rebound or guarding. What diagnostic tests would be LEAST helpful in diagnosing her condition?
    (A) CBC
    (B) ESR
    (C) Colonoscopy
    (D) ERCP
    (E) Upper endoscopy

132. A 65-year-old female presents to her PCP with the complaint of a painful rash along her left flank. She notes that she had a tingling and uncomfortable sensation in the area for a couple of days before the onset of the rash. She denies any changes to medications and has otherwise felt well. Examination reveals a vesicular erythematous rash along the left flank. The right side of the trunk is unaffected. What is the most likely diagnosis?
    (A) Viral exanthema
    (B) Atopic dermatitis
    (C) Herpes zoster
    (D) Herpes simplex
    (E) Tinea Corporis

133. A patient is diagnosed with left ventricular heart failure. Which of the following types of medication is the most appropriate intervention for this condition?
    (A) Calcium channel blockers
    (B) Beta blockers
    (C) Clopidogrel (Plavix)
    (D) ACE inhibitors
    (E) Digoxin

134. Which of the following is an effective treatment for chronic thrombocytopenia?
    (A) Vitamin B_{12}
    (B) Folic acid
    (C) Vitamin D
    (D) Prednisone
    (E) Erythropoietin

135. A patient suffering from conversion disorder can be most effectively treated with which of the following medications?
    (A) Tricyclic antidepressants
    (B) Antipsychotic medications
    (C) SSRIs
    (D) MAOIs
    (E) None of the above

136. A 73-year-old Caucasian male with hypertension, hyperlipidemia, and 50 packs/year history of smoking presents with a chief complaint of decreased visual acuity on reading, which has been gradual. He also complains of a blind spot in his center of vision. Which of the following is the most appropriate diagnosis?
    (A) Uveitis
    (B) Macular degeneration
    (C) Cataract
    (D) Glaucoma
    (E) Retinal detachment

137. Which of the following is the proper treatment for individuals with achalasia?
    (A) Metoclopramide (Reglan)
    (B) Gastropexy
    (C) Esophagoduodenoscopy with dilation (EGD)
    (D) Proton pump inhibitors (PPI)
    (E) Histamine antagonists (H_2 blocker)

138. A 2-year-old presents to her PCP with meningitis. What is the most likely bacterial etiology?
    (A) *Neisseria meningitidis*
    (B) *Streptococcus pneumoniae*
    (C) *Staphylococcus aureus*
    (D) *Mycobacterium tuberculosis*
    (E) *Haemophilus influenza*

139. A 35-year-old female presents to her PCP with complaints of excessive sweating, palpitations, weight loss, and tremor. Examination reveals BP 150/80. Neck is supple with diffuse enlargement of the thyroid gland. What is the most likely diagnosis?
    (A) Anxiety
    (B) Pheochromocytoma
    (C) Hyperthyroidism
    (D) Menopause
    (E) Anxiety

140. A 12-year-old female presents to her PCP with the complaint of wheezing and coughing when running during soccer. Examination reveals scattered wheezes throughout all lung fields. Which of the following is NOT an appropriate diagnostic tool?
    (A) Spirometry
    (B) CT scan
    (C) Chest X-ray
    (D) Peak expiratory flow meter
    (E) Both (B) and (D)

141. Spina bifida is also known as a myelomeningocele. This defect occurs when the caudal end of the neural tube fails to close. This causes a protrusion of the spinal cord through the defect. How can this defect most effectively be avoided?
    (A) Vaccination
    (B) Antibiotic therapy
    (C) Ingestion of B_9 (folic acid) supplements before and during pregnancy
    (D) Exercise
    (E) Limit the amount of glucose during pregnancy

142. All of the following are important diagnostic tools in diagnosing the etiology of chronic cough in an adult EXCEPT
    (A) PPD
    (B) Chest X-ray
    (C) Spirometry
    (D) Sweat chloride test
    (E) 24-hour pH probe

143. A 6-year-old girl presents with hair growth in the axilla, accelerated growth, and menarche. She also has been exhibiting uncharacteristic behavior at school. Which of the following is the most appropriate diagnosis?
    (A) Lupus
    (B) Hyperthyroidism
    (C) Turner syndrome
    (D) Acromegaly
    (E) Precocious puberty

144. A 3-year-old boy presents with his mother at the emergency room with the complaint of fever, sore throat, and drooling. Examination reveals a toxic-appearing child who is sitting and leaning forward with his head extended, jaw thrust forward, and drooling. Which of the following is NOT an appropriate diagnostic tool?
    (A) Examination with tongue depressor
    (B) Lateral neck X-ray
    (C) CBC
    (D) Blood cultures
    (E) Vital signs.

145. A Snellen Chart may be used in the evaluation of eye trauma to assess which of the following?
    (A) Intraocular pressure
    (B) Corneal abrasions
    (C) Pupillary reactions
    (D) Visual acuity
    (E) Peripheral vision

146. A 65-year-old male presents to his PCP for a routine physical with complaints of fatigue, constipation, and mucus in the stool. Examination reveals heme positive stool but is otherwise negative. However, CBC reveals a HgB of 10.2 g/dl and an MCV of 68. What is the most likely diagnosis?
    (A) Peptic ulcer disease
    (B) Ulcerative colitis
    (C) Diverticulitis
    (D) Colon cancer
    (E) Crohn's disease

147. A 70-year-old female with diabetes and CHF presents to her PCP complaining of fatigue and "racing heart beat." Examination reveals BP 150/80. Pulse is irregularly irregular at 170 bpm. Cardiac exam reveals tachycardia and an irregularly irregular rhythm. EKG shows tachycardia, left axis deviation, and a wavy baseline with no defined P wave. Which of the following is NOT an appropriate intervention for this patient?
    (A) Beta-blockers
    (B) Aspirin
    (C) Heparin
    (D) Immediate cardioversion
    (E) Diltiazem

148. Sildenafil is commonly used to treat which of the following disorders?
    (A) Schizophrenia
    (B) Erectile dysfunction
    (C) Pelvic inflammatory disease
    (D) Chronic obstructive pulmonary disease
    (E) Tuberculosis

149. A 65-year-old woman with hypertension presents to the emergency room after experiencing weakness and paresthesias in the left arm that lasted for 20 minutes. Current medications include hydrochlorothiazide. Examination reveals a II/VI systolic murmur heard loudest at the apex, a normal neurologic exam, and a BP of 130/80. Non-contrast CT of the brain is negative for ischemia. Which of the following medications is most appropriate?
    (A) Antibiotics
    (B) Anticonvulsants
    (C) Antidepressants
    (D) Aspirin
    (E) Increase dosage of current medication

150. Which of the following refers to a psychiatric disorder in which individuals intentionally inflict or create the symptoms of an illness?
    (A) Borderline personality disorder
    (B) Schizophrenia
    (C) Pain disorder
    (D) Malingering
    (E) Hypochondriasis

151. A 35-year-old male presents to his PCP with the complaint of scaling greasy plaques around the eyebrows and scalp. Examination reveals erythema and greasy scales around the margin of the scalp and eyebrows. Otherwise, examination is normal. What is the most effective treatment plan?
    (A) Ketoconazole shampoo
    (B) High potency steroid cream
    (C) Bactroban ointment
    (D) Reassurance
    (E) None of the above

152. A 65-year-old male with a 60 packs/year history of smoking and hypertension presents with complaints of non-productive cough. Physical examination reveals BP 130/80. Pharynx is pink, moist, and without exudate. Cardiac and pulmonary exams are normal. What is the most appropriate FIRST step?
    (A) Upper endoscopy
    (B) Referral to ENT
    (C) Chest X-ray
    (D) Medication review
    (E) EKG

153. Which of the following is commonly used in conjunction with antihistamines for the treatment of mild atopic dermatitis?
    (A) Prednisolone
    (B) Topical corticosteroids
    (C) Cyclosporine
    (D) Tacrolimus
    (E) Prednisone

154. A 25-year-old female presents with a chief complaint of irregular menstrual periods. Physical exam is significant for BP of 150/80, acne, hirsuitism, a buffalo hump, moon facies, and telangectasias. A urinalysis reveals 2+ glucose. Further testing reveals an elevated 24-hour urine cortisol. Which of the following is the most appropriate diagnosis?
(A) Polycystic ovary syndrome
(B) Diabetes mellitus
(C) Addison's disease
(D) Cushing's disease
(E) Hashimoto's disease

155. A 45-year-old male presents to the emergency room by ambulance with his wife. He complains of racing heart beat and weakness that started in the legs and seems to be "creeping up my body." Shortly before presenting to the emergency room, he had a syncopal episode and shortness of breath. Past medical history is significant only for a recent "stomach bug" that started after a vacation overseas. Physical exam reveals 0/5 ankle jerk reflex and hypotension. Which of the following is the most common group of tests ordered to diagnose his disease?
(A) Holter monitoring / Nerve conduction study (NCS) / Pulmonary function test
(B) Lumbar puncture for cerebrospinal fluid (CSF) / Electromyography (EMG) / Nerve conduction study (NCS)
(C) Electrocardiogram (ECG) / Complete blood count (CBC) / Lumbar puncture for cerebrospinal fluid (CSF)
(D) Nerve conduction study / Arthrocentesis / Electromyography (EMG)
(E) Pulmonary function test / Electroencephalography (EEG) / Electrocardiogram (ECG)

156. A 23-year-old female presents to her PCP with the complaint of progressive hearing loss in the right ear over the past year. She denies vertigo or tinnitus. Family history is significant for early hearing loss. Examination reveals a normal TM and external ear canal. Nasal mucosa is pink and moist. Pharynx is without exudate or erythema, 1+ tonsils. Weber's test lateralizes to the right ear. What is the most likely diagnosis?
(A) Serous otitis media
(B) Acoustic neuroma
(C) Cerumen impaction
(D) Otosclerosis
(E) Presbycusis

157. Which of the following refers to osteochondrosis of the tibial tubercle?
(A) Werdnig-Hoffmann disease
(B) Osgood-Schlatter disease
(C) Eagle-Barrett syndrome
(D) Wernicke-Korsakoff syndrome
(E) Osler's disease

158. Which of the following medications would be the most appropriate for the treatment of individuals with hypertriglyceridemia?
(A) Lovastatin (Mevacor)
(B) Niacin (Niaspan)
(C) Gemfibrozil (Lopid)
(D) Colestipol (Colestid)
(E) Fluvastatin (Lescol)

159. A 42-year-old male presents to his PCP with complaints of urinary frequency for about two weeks. He also notes a low-grade fever and pain in the perineum. He is married and denies any extramarital affairs. Examination reveals an enlarged boggy prostate. Urinalysis is negative. What is the most likely diagnosis?
(A) Urinary tract infection
(B) Benign prostatic hypertrophy
(C) Prostatitis
(D) Nephrolithiasis
(E) Gonococcal urethritis

160. Which of the following refers to coronary artery spasm that occurs while the patient is at rest?
    (A) Syndrome X
    (B) Stable angina
    (C) Thrombocytosis
    (D) Unstable angina
    (E) Variant angina

161. Risperidone is commonly used to treat which of the following disorders?
    (A) Borderline personality disorder
    (B) Schizophrenia
    (C) Depression
    (D) Conversion disorder
    (E) Body dysmorphic disorder

162. The HPV vaccine is commonly administered to prevent which of the following disorders?
    (A) Ovarian cancer
    (B) Swine flu
    (C) Prostate cancer
    (D) Cervical cancer
    (E) Paget's disease

163. Which of the following is a gram-positive bacilli?
    (A) *Staphylococcus aureus*
    (B) *Bacteroides fragilis*
    (C) *Bordetella pertussis*
    (D) *Clostridium difficile*
    (E) *Neisseria meningitides*

164. A 55-year-old African American male with a 30 packs/year history of smoking presents to his PCP with a complaint of swelling in the right lower leg. The patient reports that he recently returned from a 15-hour road trip from New York, which he proudly states he made in a "straight shot." On examination, his BP is 140/90. Cardiac and pulmonary examinations are essentially normal. Examination of the extremities reveals 2+ pitting edema in the right leg and positive "Homan's sign." What is the most appropriate next test to order in this patient?
    (A) Arterial flow studies
    (B) Venous Doppler
    (C) CBC
    (D) EKG
    (E) Chest X-ray

165. A 57-year-old male with HTN and a 50 packs/year smoking history presents to his PCP with a complaint of intermittent "cramps" in his left leg. He works for the local cable company and his job includes quite a bit of walking. The pain in his left leg starts after walking about 50 feet. He states that he first noticed the pain about six months ago, but, at that time, he could walk at least a mile before the "cramp" began. The pain resolves with rest. Which of the following is NOT appropriate management of the patient's condition?
    (A) Initiate ASA therapy
    (B) Cyclobenzaprine 10 mg
    (C) Arterial flow studies
    (D) EKG
    (E) MI risk stratification

166. A 25-year-old male presents to the emergency room with severe pain in the right flank that radiates to the groin, nausea, and vomiting. Examination reveals a well-developed male in acute distress, with tachycardia and CVA tenderness. He does not have rebound or guarding. Rectal examination is negative for occult blood. Urinalysis reveals 3+ blood. What is the most likely diagnosis?
    (A) Appendicitis
    (B) Nephrolithiasis
    (C) Prostatitis
    (D) Diverticulitis
    (E) Peptic ulcer disease

167. A 25-year-old female with a recent history of mononucleosis that resolved last week presents with a non-pruritic rash that started the day before. Examination reveals multiple target lesions of various sizes. The rash is primarily limited to the extensor surfaces of the arms and legs. What is the most likely diagnosis?
    (A) Secondary syphilis
    (B) Viral exanthem
    (C) Herpes simplex
    (D) Erythema multiforme
    (E) Chicken pox

168. Which of the following type of bacteria is the most common cause of Rocky Mountain Spotted Fever?
    (A) *Citrobacter diversus*
    (B) *Bacillus cereus*
    (C) *Borrelia burgdorferi*
    (D) *Rickettsia rickettsii*
    (E) *Enterobacteriaceae*

169. Which of the following medications is one of the first lines of treatment for stable angina pectoris?
(A) Amiodarone
(B) Lopressor
(C) Lovastatin
(D) Lovenox
(E) Digoxin

170. A 54-year-old male with diabetes presents to his PCP for a regular physical. He complains of a "trigger finger." After working on his car, he often has a finger that stays bent and straightens with a "pop." Examination is essentially normal; however, he demonstrates the popping of the "trigger finger." What is the most likely diagnosis?
(A) Stenosing tenosynovitis
(B) Rheumatoid arthritis
(C) Osteoarthritis
(D) Gouty arthritis
(E) None of the above

171. Which of the following is the drug of choice for the prevention of pulmonary embolism?
(A) ACE inhibitors
(B) Heparin
(C) Streptokinase
(D) Beta-blockers
(E) Ciprofloxacin

172. Diabetes insipidus that occurs during pregnancy is most effectively treated by which of the following medications?
(A) Ergocalciferol
(B) Desmopressin acetate
(C) Lovastatin
(D) Vancomycin
(E) Metronidazole

173. Each of the following is a prevalent cause of blindness EXCEPT
(A) Diabetic retinopathy
(B) Cataracts
(C) Glaucoma
(D) Macular degeneration
(E) Blepharitis

174. A 55-year-old female presents to the emergency room complaining of fever, chills, and pain in the right flank. She was treated two weeks ago for a urinary tract infection with three days of Bactrim. Examination reveals a temperature of 38.7°C. She is tachycardic and has CVA tenderness on the right side. Urinalysis reveals 3+ Leukocytes, 3+ blood, and 1+ protein. What is the most likely diagnosis?
(A) Urinary tract infection
(B) Pyelonephritis
(C) Nephrolithiasis
(D) Pelvic inflammatory disease
(E) Ectopic pregnancy

175. Which of the following is most common etiology of ischemic heart disease?
(A) Congenital defect
(B) Atherosclerosis
(C) Adenovirus
(D) Valvular heart diseases
(E) Embolism

176. Which of the following is a cyanotic type of congenital heart defect?
(A) Patent ductus arteriosus
(B) Atrioventricular septal defect
(C) Atrial septal defect
(D) Truncus arteriosus
(E) Ventricular septal defect

177. A 65-year-old male presents to his PCP with his daughter. She states that the patient has had a tremor that is mostly noticed at rest. The tremor started in one hand but seems to be worsening and becoming more pervasive. The daughter also states that the patient has been confused and "moody" and has been having difficulty eating and speaking. Examination reveals cogwheel rigidity of the limbs and bradykinesia. What is the most appropriate treatment for this patient's condition?
(A) Rimantadine (Flumadine)
(B) Levodopa-Carbidopa (Sinemet)
(C) Fluoxetine (Prozac)
(D) Valproic acid (Depakene)
(E) Carbamazepine (Tegretol)

178. Metoclopramide is commonly prescribed in the treatment of which of the following disorders?
    (A) Rheumatoid arthritis
    (B) Asthma
    (C) Gastroparesis
    (D) Osteoarthritis
    (E) Gout

179. A 55-year-old male with a long history of alcoholism presents to the emergency room complaining of dyspnea on exertion, lower extremity edema, and orthopnea. Examination reveals jugular venous distention, a III/VI systolic murmur heard loudest at the apex, bibasilar rales, hepatomegaly, and 3+ pedal edema. What is the most likely diagnosis?
    (A) Restrictive cardiomyopathy
    (B) Dilated cardiomyopathy
    (C) Hypertrophic cardiomyopathy
    (D) Cor pumonale
    (E) Pulmonary hypertension

180. Dermatophytes can be effectively identified using which of the following diagnostic procedures?
    (A) Patch test
    (B) Immunofluorescence
    (C) KOH prep
    (D) Doppler study
    (E) Acetowhitening

181. Albendazole is commonly used to treat which of the following disorders?
    (A) Cryptosporidiosis
    (B) Demodicosis
    (C) Ascariasis
    (D) Aspergillosis
    (E) Neurocysticercosis

182. In which of the following juvenile onset disorders do patients typically display high fever and a characteristic rash?
    (A) Osteoarthritis
    (B) Amblyopia
    (C) Still's disease
    (D) Tay-Sachs disease
    (E) Polymyositis

183. Increasing the intake of fluids and dietary sodium can help to treat which of the following?
    (A) Congestive heart failure
    (B) Essential hypertension
    (C) Orthostatic hypotension
    (D) Pulmonary hypertension
    (E) Diabetes mellitus

184. A 75-year-old African American female who has been living in a senior home care facility for more than a year is brought to the clinic by her nurse to be evaluated. The nurse states that the patient is not able to carry out her normal daily activities. She also notes that the patient has a flat affect and decreased interest in activities that she normally enjoys. The nurse states that the patient has become anxious and is having difficulty remembering things that happened recently. The nurse states that the patient did not seem to know her daughter at the last visitation period. Which of the following medications would be helpful in delaying the deterioration of cognition in this patient?
    (A) Oxazepam (Serax)
    (B) Citalopram (Celexa)
    (C) Clozapine (Clozaril)
    (D) Rivastigmine (Exelon)
    (E) Lorazepam (Ativan)

185. A 35-year-old HIV-positive male who has been non-compliant with his treatment regimen presents to the emergency room with the complaint of dyspnea, fatigue, fever, and non-productive cough. Chest X-ray is normal. What is the most likely diagnosis?
    (A) Tuberculosis
    (B) *Pneumocystis carinii* pneumonia
    (C) Bronchitis
    (D) Pneumonia due to *Streptococcus pneumoniae*
    (E) *Mycobacterium avium* complex

186. A 3-year-old boy presents with his mother to the ER with complaints of sore throat, fever, and drooling that came on very suddenly. His mother reports that he is not up-to-date on vaccinations. Examination reveals a febrile, well-nourished male who is sitting propped up on his hands with his tongue sticking out. What is the NEXT most important step in treating this patient?
    (A) Keep patient quiet while preparing for intubation
    (B) Lateral neck X-ray
    (C) Blood culture
    (D) Rapid strep test
    (E) Visualization of pharynx with a tongue depressor

187. Which of the following is an effective treatment for chronic thrombocytopenia?
(A) Vitamin B_{12}
(B) Folic acid
(C) Vitamin D
(D) Prednisone
(E) Erythropoietin

188. Which of the following side effects is a risk associated with taking Risperidone?
(A) Vaginal yeast infection
(B) Hyponatremia
(C) Hypokalemia
(D) Urinary tract infection
(E) Metabolic syndrome

189. A 21-year-old male presents after head trauma with frequent urination and craving for ice water. Urinalysis reveals a specific gravity of 1.002 with an osmolality of 184 mOsm/Kg H2O. The vasopressin challenge test is positive. Which of the following is the most accurate diagnosis?
(A) Addison's disease
(B) Cushing's disease
(C) Acromegaly
(D) Grave's disease
(E) Diabetes insipidus

190. Photodynamic therapy (PDT) is the procedure performed in order to correct which of the following disorders?
(A) Barrett's esophagus
(B) Achalasia
(C) Mallory-Weiss tear
(D) Pyloric stenosis
(E) Esophageal atresia

191. A 57-year-old female with known coronary artery disease presents to her PCP for a regular physical. She states that since an MI three years ago, she has retrosternal chest pain radiating to the jaw that lasts for 5 minutes and is alleviated by rest and nitroglycerine. She always has the pain when walking up the steps to her office. She denies any lower extremity edema, cough, orthopnea, nausea, or vomiting. Examination is unchanged from her last visit. What is the most likely diagnosis?
(A) Stable angina
(B) Costochondritis
(C) Gastroesophageal reflux disease
(D) Pericarditis
(E) Myocarditis

192. Which of the following medications is NOT an effective treatment for shigellosis?
(A) TMP/SMX
(B) Ciprofloxacin
(C) Levofloxacin
(D) Ampicillin
(E) Norfloxacin

193. A 7-year-old boy has fallen from a tree and has a severe deformity of the forearm proximal to the wrist. He has fractured the radius and the ulna (Monteggia fracture), and the fracture is unstable. Which of the following is the proper treatment?
(A) Traction
(B) Surgery
(C) Splint
(D) Cast
(E) Manual manipulation

194. A 55-year-old woman with diabetes presents with pain in the right ear associated with drainage. Examination reveals an occluded ear canal with purulent drainage. What is the most likely etiology of the infection?
(A) *Staphylococcus*
(B) *Streptococcus*
(C) *Pseudomonas*
(D) Fungi
(E) None of the above

195. A 37-year-old male patient is found to have osteomyelitis due to *Pseudomonas aeruginosa*. Which of the following medications is appropriate for treating this condition?
(A) Penicillin G
(B) Ampicillin
(C) Amoxicillin
(D) Cefuroxime
(E) Cefepime

196. Each of the following medications could be prescribed to effectively treat generalized anxiety disorder, EXCEPT
(A) Sertraline (Zoloft)
(B) Paroxetine (Paxil)
(C) Haloperidol (Haldol)
(D) Fluoxetine (Prozac)
(E) Escitalopram (Lexipro)

197. A 35-year-old female presents to the emergency room with signs and symptoms suggestive of pancreatitis. She denies a history of heavy drinking. Which of the following tests will NOT help to conclude the etiology of her condition?
 (A) Lipid profile
 (B) Gallblader ultrasound
 (C) Colonoscopy
 (D) Autoimmune profile
 (E) CT of abdomen

198. A 16-year-old Hispanic obese male presents with polydipsia, decreased visual acuity, and fatigue. His mother states that he has been losing a noticeable amount of weight lately but has still been eating the same amount of food as usual. A random plasma glucose level was measured at 220 mg/dL. Based on the patient's presentation and lab results, which of the following is the most accurate diagnosis?
 (A) Grave's disease
 (B) Diabetes insipidus
 (C) Addison's disease
 (D) Diabetes mellitus Type I
 (E) Diabetes mellitus Type II

199. A 45-year-old male presents to the ER after experiencing chest pain and dyspnea. EKG shows a prominent S wave in lead 1 and a Q wave and inverted T wave in lead 3. What is the most important NEXT test?
 (A) Troponin
 (B) CT of chest
 (C) CBC
 (D) CMP
 (E) Sputum culture

200. A 71-year-old male presents with advanced cirrhosis, caput medusa, prominent ascites, subicteric skin, and sclera. He also complains of nausea and vomiting. Which of the following procedures is relatively contraindicated for this condition?
 (A) Abdominal ultrasound
 (B) Esophagogastroduodenoscopy (EGD)
 (C) Laparocentesis
 (D) Graham-Cole test
 (E) Magnetic resonance imaging (MRI)

201. A 57-year-old male with a 50 packs/year history of smoking presents to his PCP with a six-month history of chronic cough. He reports that the cough is productive in nature and frequently associated with wheezing. Examination of the chest reveals scattered rhonchi and wheezes. Heart sounds are diminished. Pulmonary function testing reveals a reduction in FEV1/FVC ratio that does not respond to bronchodilators. What is the most likely diagnosis?
 (A) Asthma
 (B) Acute bronchitis
 (C) Chronic obstructive pulmonary disease
 (D) Bronchiectasis
 (E) Smoker's cough

202. A 3-year-old female presents with her mother who states that the child has appeared pale for several weeks. Five days ago, she developed a low-grade fever and has been complaining of various aches and pains. CBC reveals a WBC of 23,000 with relative neutropenia, Hgb of 8.2 g/dL, and platelets of 90,000. Peripheral smear reveals lymphoblasts. What is the most likely diagnosis?
 (A) Aplastic anemia
 (B) Acute lymphoblastic leukemia
 (C) Lupus
 (D) Mononucleosis
 (E) Viral syndrome

203. A spot urine test uses a sample size of which of the following?
 (A) 10–20 mL
 (B) 40–50 mL
 (C) 45–60 mL
 (D) 90–100 mL
 (E) 120–150 mL

204. Which of the following is suspected in an adult with slipped capital femoral epiphysis?
 (A) Hyperkalemia
 (B) Multiple sclerosis
 (C) Meningitis
 (D) Rheumatoid arthritis
 (E) Hypothyroidism

205. A 55-year-old female presents to her PCP complaining of progressive fatigue, vague abdominal pain, and mild nausea. This has been going on for 5 years or more, but she has attributed it to "getting older." Family history is essentially negative. Both her parents are living and well in their eighties. Past medical history is negative except for a blood transfusion after the birth of her first child in 1980. Laboratory examination reveals an ALT of 310 U/L and AST of 250 U/L. Alkaline phosphatase is 252 U/L. What is the most important next test?

(A) CT abdomen
(B) Colonoscopy
(C) Viral hepatitis profile
(D) HIV test
(E) Abdominal ultrasound

206. A 65-year-old female presents to the emergency room with complaints of dyspnea on exertion, orthopnea, and bilateral lower extremity edema. Examination reveals a chronically ill appearing female whose head bobs rhythmically. PMI is laterally displaced and enlarged. There is a high-pitched blowing decrescendo murmur heard in diastole and loudest at the left sternal border. What is the most likely diagnosis?

(A) Aortic stenosis
(B) Aortic regurgitation
(C) Mitral regurgitation
(D) Mitral stenosis
(E) Tricuspid regurgitation

207. Which of the following medications is administered as an antidote in the treatment of morphine overdose?

(A) Protamine
(B) Sodium bicarbonate
(C) Flumazenil
(D) Phenobarbitol
(E) Naloxone

208. Which of the following test results would suggest conductive hearing loss in the right ear? (Note: AC = air conduction, BC = bone conduction.)

(A) Weber test lateralizes to the left ear, Rinne test reveals AC>BC on the right
(B) Weber test lateralizes to the right ear, Rinne test reveals AC>BC on the right
(C) Weber test lateralizes to the right ear, Rinne test reveals BC>AC on the right
(D) Weber test lateralizes to the left ear, Rinne test reveals BC>AC on the right
(E) Weber test lateralizes to the left ear, Rinne test reveals BC>AC on the left

209. A 45-year-old female with systemic lupus erythematosus presents for a routine check-up. Examination reveals a IV/VI systolic blowing holosystolic murmur that radiates to the axilla. There is a thrill palpated at the apex. What is the most likely diagnosis?

(A) Aortic stenosis
(B) Mitral regurgitation
(C) Mitral stenosis
(D) Tricuspid regurgitation
(E) Aortic regurgitation

210. A 42-year-old obese male presents to his PCP with the complaint of excessive fatigue and headache. He states that he even feels tired upon waking and can even fall asleep while waiting at traffic lights. Examination reveals an obese male with a neck circumference of 19 inches. Visualization of the tonsilar pillars and uvula is not possible without using a tongue depressor. What is the most important diagnostic tool in evaluating this patient?

(A) CT of brain
(B) Overnight oximetry
(C) CBC
(D) TSH
(E) Lateral neck X-ray

211. Which of the following is an appropriate treatment for rubella virus?

(A) Acyclovir
(B) Ganciclovir
(C) Acetaminophen
(D) Rimantadine
(E) Amantadine

212. A 15-year-old boy with a history of attention deficit hyperactivity disorder (ADHD) presents to his PCP with a two-week history of nodding, clapping hands, throat clearing, and inappropriate vocal outbursts. His mother states that the symptoms seem to worsen when he is under stress. Which of the following is the most likely diagnosis?

(A) Neuroacanthocytosis
(B) Complex partial seizures
(C) Hemifacial spasm
(D) Tourette syndrome
(E) Huntington's disease

213. A patient presents to his PCP with suspected peripheral arterial disease. After physical exam, what is the most important next test to confirm this diagnosis?
    (A) Arterial flow studies
    (B) X-ray
    (C) Venous Doppler
    (D) D-Dimer
    (E) None of the above

214. A 55-year-old female presents to her PCP with complaints of decreased hearing and fullness in the right ear. The patient acknowledges a smoking history but denies any prior history of ear infections and has otherwise felt well. Examination reveals a dull tympanic membrane with loss of bony landmarks and an amber fluid behind the TM. The left ear is normal. What is the most appropriate next step?
    (A) Audiogram
    (B) Tympanogram
    (C) Amoxicillan
    (D) Nasopharyngoscopy
    (E) Culture of middle ear fluid

215. Lithium is commonly used to treat which of the following?
    (A) Seizure disorder
    (B) Anorexia
    (C) Bipolar disorder Type 1
    (D) Schizophrenia
    (E) Depression

216. Which of the following types of medications is the most appropriate intervention in conjunction with nitroglycerin for conditions related to coronary artery spasms?
    (A) Angiotensin-converting enzyme (ACE) inhibitors
    (B) Anticoagulants
    (C) Antiarrhythmic medications
    (D) Calcium channel blockers
    (E) Diuretics

217. Which of the following modalities would be used to confirm the diagnosis of a Mallory-Weiss tear?
    (A) MRI
    (B) Urea breath test
    (C) Pulmonary angiography
    (D) Percutaneous transhepatic cholangiography
    (E) Endoscopy

218. A 75-year-old woman with multi-infarct dementia presents to the emergency room with her daughter. Her daughter complains that the patient has been more confused for the past three days and has become increasingly disoriented. She also suffers from frequent urinary tract infections and was treated for one a month ago with three days of Bactrim. The patient is uncooperative and combative on examination. What is the most likely diagnosis?
    (A) Acute psychotic episode
    (B) Dissociative disorder
    (C) Adjustment disorder
    (D) Posttraumatic stress disorder
    (E) Delirium

219. A 52-year-old female presents to the emergency room with a complaint of epigastric pain that is brought on by eating. She has experienced some relief with OTC antacids. Examination reveals a diffusely tender epigastrium without rebound or guarding. Murphy's sign is negative. What is the most specific diagnostic tool available to help diagnose this patient?
    (A) Barium swallow
    (B) Upper endoscopy
    (C) Lower endoscopy
    (D) *H. pylori* blood test
    (E) Laparotomy

220. A 35-year-old male presents to the emergency room with a headache. The patient states that he has been getting these headaches daily for the past three weeks. He reports having similar symptoms a year ago. The pain is described as retro-orbital, unilateral, and 9/10 intensity. Examination reveals erythema of the conjunctiva, lacrimation, and ptosis of the right eye. What is the most likely diagnosis?
    (A) Intracranial hemorrhage
    (B) Trigeminal neuralgia
    (C) Cluster headache
    (D) Persistent idiopathic facial pain
    (E) Subarachnoid hemorrhage

221. A 65-year-old male presents to his PCP with complaints of an exquisitely painful right knee. He drinks beer daily and lately has been drinking more and eating more red meat. Which of the following is the MOST specific diagnostic tool to confirm this condition?
  (A) Arthrocentesis
  (B) X-ray
  (C) Uric acid level
  (D) Rheumatoid factor
  (E) ESR

222. A 60-year-old male presents to his PCP for a routine physical. Current medications include Atenolol 50 mg and HCTZ 12.5 mg. He has a 40 packs/year history of smoking. Examination reveals a pulsatile mass in the epigastrium. What is the most important NEXT step?
  (A) GI consult
  (B) Urinalysis
  (C) CT scan
  (D) Nasogastric tube
  (E) Consult about tobacco cessation

223. A 19-year-old male presents to the emergency room after getting in a fight at a hockey game. He is complaining of pain in his right hand. Examination reveals tenderness over the knuckles. What is the most likely diagnosis?
  (A) Fracture of the radius
  (B) Fracture of the first distal phalynx
  (C) Fracture of the fifth metacarpal
  (D) Fracture of the lunate
  (E) None of the above

224. A 30-year-old woman with a history of epilepsy adequately treated with phenytoin presents to her PCP with her husband because she has been having trouble walking and speaking. Her gums are swollen, and she states that they bleed very easily when she brushes her teeth. There is no history of alcohol or illicit drug use. Physical examination reveals gingival hyperplasia, dysarthria, and ataxia. What is the most likely cause of this condition?
  (A) Infection
  (B) Depression
  (C) Psychotic state
  (D) Adverse reaction to phenytoin
  (E) Partial seizure

225. A 26-year-old female with a three-year history of depression presents to her PCP with her mother. She has recently been in jail for shoplifting and has had multiple D.U.I. arrests. She has been treated with multiple SSRI medications in the past, which were not effective. Further questioning reveals that she often has periods where she is "on top of the world." During these times, she has an abnormal amount of energy where she can "do anything." Her mother reports that during these episodes, she frequently steals her credit cards and will disappear for days. After these episodes she will have periods of time where she will not leave her room and is very lethargic. Her mother states that this has been her behavior since her teen years, but recently it has worsened. What is the most likely diagnosis?
  (A) Depression with psychotic features
  (B) Bipolar disorder
  (C) Schizophrenia
  (D) Drug abuse
  (E) ADHD

226. A 20-year-old female presents to the emergency room with the complaint of pelvic pain, vaginal bleeding, and nausea. Physical exam reveals an adenexal mass on the right. Which of the following diagnostic modalities is the LEAST appropriate?
  (A) Quantitative Beta hCG
  (B) Pelvic ultrasound
  (C) Pap and HPV
  (D) GC/chlamydia
  (E) None of the above

227. A patient will be receiving oxygen for a prolonged period of time. Which of the following modalities should be put into place for this patient?
  (A) Set flow rate at <4 L/min
  (B) Oxygen humidifier
  (C) Nasal cannula is all that is necessary
  (D) Take hourly breaks from oxygen
  (E) Hyperbaric oxygen treatments

228. Which of the following is an effective treatment for chronic thrombocytopenia?
  (A) Vitamin B_{12}
  (B) Folic acid
  (C) Vitamin D
  (D) Prednisone
  (E) Erythropoietin

229. A 20-year-old female presents to the emergency room with syncope. There is a strong family history of sudden cardiac death. Examination is unremarkable. Which of the following is the most appropriate management of this patient?
    (A) EKG, Holter monitor, and referral to cardiology
    (B) EKG, cardiac stress test, beta-blocker
    (C) Rest, hydration, reassurance
    (D) EKG, chest X-ray, drug screen
    (E) None of the above

230. Which of the following medications is an appropriate treatment for empyema?
    (A) Meloxicam
    (B) Heparin
    (C) Penicillin
    (D) Ketoconazole
    (E) Prednisone

231. A 42-year-old male presents to the emergency room with productive cough, fever, fatigue and pleuritic chest pain. Examination reveals rales over the right lower lobe. WBC is 16,000. Gram's stain of sputum reveals gram positive diplococci. What is the most likely diagnosis?
    (A) Pneumonia due to Streptococcus pneumoniae
    (B) Congestive heart failure
    (C) Bronchitis
    (D) Pneumonia due to Haemophilus influenza
    (E) Pulmonary embolus

232. Which of the following is most important in the treatment and diagnosis of most low back pain?
    (A) Lumbar X-ray
    (B) MRI
    (C) CT
    (D) History and physical
    (E) Bone scan

233. Giardiasis is commonly treated by which of the following medications?
    (A) Mebendazole
    (B) Quinine
    (C) Lindane
    (D) Metronidazole
    (E) Miconazole

234. A 12-year-old male with a history of asthma presents to his PCP with complaints of sinus congestion, runny nose, and facial pain. Physical examination reveals a mostly occluded nasal cavity on the right side because of obstruction by large grapelike masses. What medication would be inappropriate to give this patient?
    (A) Amoxicillan
    (B) ASA
    (C) Clarithromycin
    (D) NSAID
    (E) Prednisone

235. A 30-year-old male with a history of IV drug use presents to the emergency room. The chart reveals that he is a "frequent flyer" with multiple requests for narcotics. Examination reveals a holosystolic murmur heard loudest at the left sternal border that increases with inspiration. Examination of the liver reveals hepatojugular reflux. What is the most likely diagnosis?
    (A) Mitral regurgitation
    (B) Tricuspid regurgitation
    (C) Aortic stenosis
    (D) Tricuspid stenosis
    (E) Mitral stenosis

236. A 25-year-old female was playing flag football and was tackled when her right leg was planted and flexed. She complains of swelling in the right knee and a feeling of "giving way." Which one of the following is NOT an appropriate diagnostic tool for this patient?
    (A) Anterior drawer test
    (B) Lachman's test
    (C) McMurray's test
    (D) Arthrocentesis
    (E) MRI of knee

237. A 27-year-old female presents with watery eyes, sneezing, stuffy nose, and sinus pressure. She says she also has an itchy throat and post-nasal drip. The patient confirms that she has a reoccurrence of these symptoms every spring. Examination reveals pale, boggy nasal mucosa and mild erythema of the posterior pharynx. Which of the following would be the most appropriate diagnosis?
   (A) Allergic rhinitis
   (B) Influenza
   (C) Acute sinusitis
   (D) Mastoiditis
   (E) Common cold

238. A 19-year-old male presents after a motor vehicle accident with dizziness, headache, and vomiting after loss of consciousness. CT scan of the brain is normal. Which of the following is the most accurate diagnosis?
   (A) Ruptured spleen
   (B) Cerebral aneurysm
   (C) Cerebrovascular accident
   (D) Concussion
   (E) Vertigo

239. A child is in need of emergency intravenous medication. The child's veins are inaccessible. What route of administration should be used to administer the medication?
   (A) Sublingual
   (B) Intramuscular
   (C) Subcutaneous
   (D) Transdermal
   (E) Intraosseous

240. A 33-year-old white female, with a previous history of hypothyroidism, presents with diplopia, paresthesia, dizziness, and fatigue. She complains of a "shock sensation" when she moves her head a certain way. A spinal tap reveals elevated immunoglobulin concentration with the presence of oligoclonal bands in the CSF. Which of the following is the most appropriate diagnosis?
   (A) Myasthenia gravis
   (B) Diabetes mellitus
   (C) Multiple sclerosis
   (D) Huntington's disease
   (E) Guillain-Barré syndrome

ANSWER KEY AND EXPLANATIONS

1. D	37. E	73. B	109. D	145. D	181. C
2. B	38. E	74. A	110. B	146. D	182. C
3. B	39. B	75. C	111. B	147. D	183. C
4. B	40. A	76. D	112. B	148. B	184. D
5. B	41. E	77. C	113. C	149. D	185. B
6. D	42. B	78. B	114. A	150. D	186. A
7. C	43. D	79. B	115. A	151. A	187. D
8. C	44. D	80. A	116. C	152. D	188. E
9. E	45. D	81. A	117. D	153. B	189. E
10. D	46. E	82. D	118. C	154. D	190. A
11. D	47. C	83. E	119. B	155. B	191. A
12. A	48. A	84. C	120. A	156. D	192. D
13. A	49. A	85. E	121. B	157. B	193. B
14. C	50. D	86. E	122. D	158. C	194. C
15. B	51. A	87. A	123. D	159. C	195. E
16. B	52. C	88. E	124. B	160. E	196. C
17. E	53. A	89. D	125. A	161. B	197. C
18. E	54. A	90. A	126. E	162. D	198. E
19. A	55. B	91. D	127. D	163. D	199. B
20. D	56. E	92. D	128. E	164. B	200. B
21. E	57. D	93. C	129. E	165. B	201. C
22. D	58. C	94. C	130. A	166. B	202. B
23. A	59. B	95. C	131. D	167. D	203. A
24. D	60. E	96. A	132. C	168. D	204. E
25. C	61. D	97. B	133. D	169. B	205. C
26. A	62. B	98. A	134. D	170. A	206. B
27. C	63. A	99. D	135. E	171. B	207. E
28. A	64. B	100. C	136. B	172. B	208. C
29. B	65. D	101. E	137. C	173. E	209. B
30. A	66. C	102. E	138. A	174. B	210. B
31. D	67. A	103. B	139. C	175. B	211. C
32. B	68. C	104. B	140. E	176. D	212. D
33. B	69. E	105. C	141. C	177. B	213. A
34. E	70. C	106. B	142. D	178. C	214. D
35. D	71. A	107. B	143. E	179. B	215. C
36. C	72. D	108. A	144. A	180. C	216. D

217. E
218. E
219. B
220. C
221. A
222. C
223. C
224. D
225. B
226. C
227. B
228. D
229. A
230. C
231. A
232. D
233. D
234. B
235. B
236. D
237. A
238. D
239. E
240. C

1. **The correct answer is (D).** Heparin is commonly administered for the prevention of deep venous thromboses, or blood clots.

2. **The correct answer is (B).** The patient is most likely suffering from cerebral palsy. Cerebral palsy is thought to be caused by a period of anoxia to the brain in the perinatal period.

3. **The correct answer is (B).** Mild intermittent asthma in this scenario could also be termed "exercise-induced asthma." Treatment for this consists of beta-agonist prn with activity.

4. **The correct answer is (B).** Chlorothiazide is a diuretic used in the treatment of hypertension. A patient being treated with chlorothiazide may require additional potassium via supplements and potassium-rich foods, such as bananas, raisins, and orange juice.

5. **The correct answer is (B).** Maintenance treatment of pernicious anemia typically involves IM administration of vitamin B_{12}. Oral administration may also be indicated. Pernicious anemia is a condition where the body cannot make intrinsic factor protein.

6. **The correct answer is (D).** Mitral stenosis is most commonly caused by a prior episode of rheumatic fever. Because of the decreased incidence of rheumatic fever, this incidence is decreasing. Mitral stenosis is caused by calcification of the leaflets. This causes left atrial dilation and pulmonary hypertension.

7. **The correct answer is (C).** Addison's disease is characterized by myalgias, arthralgias, nausea, and vomiting along with hypotension. The adrenocorticotropic hormone (ACTH) stimulation test is a definitive test for diagnosing and quantifying adrenal insufficiency and Addison's disease. A patient with adrenal insufficiency will have a baseline around 15 µg/dL. A patient with Addison's disease will have a cortisol level of 10 µg/dl. The response to ACTH stimulation will be no more than 25 percent.

8. **The correct answer is (C).** Braxton Hicks contractions are mild contractions that occur after the sixth week of pregnancy but do not signal the start of labor. They were named for the doctor, John Braxton Hicks, who originally described them.

9. **The correct answer is (E).** All of the above are appropriate interventions for a patient experiencing chest pain. Morphine both controls pain and lowers blood pressure. Oxygen is important, although recent studies show that it is important not to over ventilate a patient due to free radical formation. Nitroglycerine relaxes cardiac smooth muscle and aspirin decreases platelet aggregation.

10. **The correct answer is (D).** Ophthalmoscopy is used to check the optic nerve for bulging. This swelling occurs when there is increased intracranial pressure. If the intracranial pressure is high, the spinal tap should be performed with extra precautions and at that point will be limited or withheld due to the high risk of herniation of the brain structures and possible fatality.

11. **The correct answer is (D).** Metronidazole is a common medication used to treat bacterial vaginosis and trichomoniasis. Even small amounts of alcohol can trigger a disulfram reaction. The patient should be counseled to abstain from alcohol during treatment and for 48 hours after cessation of the medication.

12. **The correct answer is (A).** Tolterodine is used to treat urinary incontinence. It is an antimuscarinic medication for the treatment of overactive bladder.

13. **The correct answer is (A).** *Cyclospora* infection is caused by the protozoan *Cyclospora* cayetanensis. TMP/SMX (trimethoprim/sulfamethoxazole) is the current drug of choice for treatment.

14. **The correct answer is (C).** Pancreatic cancer often presents with the triad of pain, weight loss, and jaundice. Risk factors include tobacco use. Men are more commonly affected than women.

15. **The correct answer is (B).** All of the answer choices are possible causes of cardiac infections. Endocarditis is the most likely diagnosis with these symptoms and the history of IV drug use. Staphylococcus aureus is the most common causative agent in patients with a history of IV drug use.

16. **The correct answer is (B).** This patient is experiencing neurologic symptoms due to thiamine deficiency. The most common cause of this vitamin deficiency in the United States is alcoholism. Patients who suffer from alcoholism often have poor eating habits, and this leads to deficiency over time. The most important first step for this patient is to assess him for alcoholism and make the appropriate referral for treatment. The thiamine deficiency can then be corrected with thiamine hydrochloride, which can be given orally or IM. Ensuring adequate oral intake of fruits, vegetables, and grains is crucially important as well.

17. **The correct answer is (E).** Scleroderma is an autoimmune disorder that affects the connective tissue. It involves a buildup of collagen, causing thickening and tightness in the skin. Systemic scleroderma, or sclerosis, may be limited or diffuse, with diffuse sclerosis affecting large areas of skin and the organs.

18. **The correct answer is (E).** Past Epstein-Barr infection is considered a risk factor for Hodgkin's lymphoma. Other risk factors include immuno-compromise and treatment with phenytoin.

19. **The correct answer is (A).** Misoprostol is a medication used to prevent the occurrence of aspirin- and NSAID-induced ulcers. It is also an abortifacient.

20. **The correct answer is (D).** Behçet syndrome is a rare disease that affects oral and genital mucosa, as well as a multi-system disease. Arthritis, uveitis, and colitis are common accompanying syndromes. Behçet syndrome is more common in people of Middle Eastern and Japanese descent.

21. **The correct answer is (E).** Sjögren's syndrome is a glandular disorder with no known etiology. The condition is characterized by dry, scaly skin (ichthyosis); neurological problems; and eye problems. These symptoms appear in early childhood, but usually do not worsen with age. Sjögren's syndrome may be primary or secondary to another autoimmune disorder.

22. **The correct answer is (D).** A photopatch test is performed to confirm the diagnosis of dermatitis that develops on skin exposed to the sun. The skin is exposed to UVA rays to determine photoallergy.

23. **The correct answer is (A).** A thyroidectomy is the only option because the high amounts of thyroid hormones are harmful for the fetus and mother if not abated. There are also limits on medication usage during pregnancy.

24. **The correct answer is (D).** Truncus arteriosus is a congential heart defect that can cause cyanosis. The remaining disorders are noncyanotic congenital defects.

25. **The correct answer is (C).** Post-traumatic stress is frequently seen in victims of severe violence and trauma. Post-traumatic stress disorder is characterized by symptoms that last for more than one month after a traumatic event, such as recurrent dreams, intrusive thoughts, and diminished interest in activities. Treatment includes psychotherapy and medications such as SSRIs.

26. **The correct answer is (A).** Individuals with chronic kidney disease should limit protein intake. Potassium and sodium may also be limited, along with other electrolytes and fluid intake.

27. **The correct answer is (C).** The presence of structural heart disease, age, and hypertension are the patient's risk factors for this condition. Other risk factors include thyroid disease, rheumatic heart disease, coronary artery disease, and past cardiac surgery.

28. **The correct answer is (A).** Trigeminal neuralgia is a poorly understood pain syndrome. The cause of the syndrome is not clear. Trigeminal neuralgia is more common in females than in males. The disease is most common in the elderly, with average age of onset between the seventh and eighth decades. The syndrome is most often unilateral. Patients tend to favor the unaffected side and avoid triggering factors.

29. **The correct answer is (B).** The most common etiologic agent for uncomplicated UTI is *E. coli*. Antibiotic therapy is indicated for both treatment and prophylaxis.

30. **The correct answer is (A).** Aortic stenosis in the elderly is commonly caused by rheumatic heart disease or calcification of the valve. Aortic stenosis can also occur congenitally. Patients can be asymptomatic. If symptomatic, most patients present with syncope, chest pain, and dyspnea.

31. **The correct answer is (D).** Antibiotics for anaerobes and gram-negative rods are the first line of treatment to eliminate the infection and the inflammation. Patients with diverticulitis should avoid consuming foods with nuts and seeds, which can become lodged in the protruding intestinal pouches.

32. **The correct answer is (B).** Sleep apnea is caused by the obstruction of the airway during sleep. The disorder is multifactorial. Risk factors include a redundant palate, large tongue, tonsil hypertrophy, and obesity. Treatment measures include the CPAP machine and, occasionally, surgery.

33. **The correct answer is (B).** Deficiency of vitamin B_{12} can lead to megaloblastic anemia. Individuals who do not consume enough meat, fish, and dairy products may develop vitamin B_{12} deficiency.

34. **The correct answer is (E).** Hordeola are typically the result of *Staphylococcus aureus* infection. The upper or lower eyelid may be affected, creating an inflamed gland or stye.

35. **The correct answer is (D).** Atopic dermatitis is a common skin condition among children. It affects both males and females equally. It is commonly associated with a history of allergies. Treatment consists of topical steroids and removal of exacerbating elements, if applicable. Oral steroids may be necessary in severe cases. In this particular patient, her condition is probably exacerbated by exposure to cold and irritating equipment like hockey gloves.

36. **The correct answer is (C).** Levothyroxine, a synthetic thyroid hormone, is used to treat hypothyroidism. Levothyroxine is contraindicated in patients with thyrotoxicosis.

37. **The correct answer is (E).** Isoniazid can be prescribed for the treatment or prevention of tuberculosis. Successful prophylaxis requires administration of the medication for periods of 6 to 12 months.

38. **The correct answer is (E).** A Gram stain is used to differentiate gram-negative from gram-positive bacteria. A Giemsa stain is used to diagnose malaria and other parasites.

39. **The correct answer is (B).** Pre-eclampsia is characterized by hypertension, proteinuria, and edema during pregnancy. Risk factors include low socioeconomic status and primigravida. Pre-eclampsia tends to occur in teenage pregnancies. Treatment is centered on decreasing seizure risk. Magnesium sulfate is given along with medications to control hypertension. Delivery of the fetus as soon as it is viable is crucial.

40. **The correct answer is (A).** Ciprofloxacin is the treatment of choice for anthrax infection, caused by the *Bacillus anthracis* bacterium. Doxycylcine may also be prescribed.

41. **The correct answer is (E).** Valproic acid is a seizure medication commonly prescribed for the treatment of petit mal seizures. Alternative treatments include ethosuximide and lamotrigine.

42. **The correct answer is (B).** Episodic vertigo, tinnitus, ear pressure, and hearing impairment are symptoms of Ménière's disease. Nausea and vomiting may also be associated.

43. **The correct answer is (D).** The patient's nasal obstruction is caused by nasal polyposis. Patients who suffer from nasal polyposis usually suffer from a triad of polyps, asthma, and ASA sensitivity.

44. **The correct answer is (D).** Addison's disease is marked by poor adrenal functioning. Addison's disease can be caused by primary dysfunction or secondary (pituitary failure). Other symptoms of Addison's disease include: changes in blood pressure or heart rate; chronic diarrhea; nausea; vomiting; or loss of appetite resulting in weight loss. Addison's disease can be confirmed by an ACTH stimulation test.

45. **The correct answer is (D).** Ceftriaxone is the preferred current medication of choice for treating gonorrhea infections. Cefixime may also be prescribed. Fluoroquinolones such as ciprofloxacin, levofloxacin, and ofloxacin were once prescribed but are no longer as effective due to the development of resistant bacterial strains.

46. **The correct answer is (E).** Obstructive sleep apnea is a sleep disorder that may worsen heart failure by reducing the flow of oxygen to the heart. The heart is required to work harder while at the same time receiving less oxygen due to narrowing of the airway during sleep.

47. **The correct answer is (C).** Siladenitis is caused by a bacterial infection of the salivary gland. Treatment consists of antibiotics and warm compresses.

48. **The correct answer is (A).** The presentation of unilateral sensorineural hearing loss is highly suspicious for acoustic neuroma. BPPV is not usually associated with hearing loss and tinnitus. Sudden sensorineural hearing loss is not usually associated with vertigo. Ménière's disease is a possibility, but the tinnitus is usually a low-pitched or "roaring" sound. Ménière's disease also presents with a characteristic low-frequency hearing loss.

49. The correct answer is (A). Ketoconazole (Nizoral) is an anti-fungal medication with adrenal-inhibiting effects. It may be administered to patients with Cushing's syndrome to help reduce cortisol production.

50. The correct answer is (D). Cobalmin (Vitamin B_{12}) deficiency, when due to pernicious anemia, results from a loss of intrinsic factor. If intrinsic factor is not produced by the gastric parietal cells, then Vitamin B_{12} cannot be absorbed in the terminal ileum. Vitamin B_{12} is necessary for proper neurologic function; deficiency causes degeneration of myelin and neuronal degeneration in the dorsal and lateral columns. This degeneration accounts for the neurologic symptoms of decreased reflexes and decreased vibratory and position sense. There is no cure for pernicious anemia, but it is easily treated with supplementation of Vitamin B_{12}.

51. The correct answer is (A). Furosemide is a loop diuretic used in the treatment of high blood pressure. Mannitol is an osmotic diuretic; triamterine and amiloride are potassium sparing diuretics; and chlorothiazide is a thiazide diuretic.

52. The correct answer is (C). Juvenile larvae of the parasite Strongyloides stercoralis can be found in the feces of the host. Diagnosis is confirmed through analysis of a stool sample.

53. The correct answer is (A). Although encephalitis can be caused by bacterial and viral infections, viral infection is more common. Herpes simplex is one of the most common causes of viral encephalitis in people over the age of 3. The incidence of herpes encephalitis is growing rapidly and is quickly becoming the most fatal sporadic cause of encephalitis in the U.S.

54. The correct answer is (A). Pleural mesothelioma is a cancer of the mesothelium of the lung. It is most commonly caused by exposure to asbestos particulate matter or dust.

55. The correct answer is (B). An ectopic pregnancy is one that forms outside the uterus. Diagnosis is confirmed by a positive beta hCG and ultrasound. Risk factors for ectopic pregnancy include pelvic inflammatory disease, use of an intrauterine device, prior pelvic surgery, and a history of endometriosis.

56. The correct answer is (E). Imatinib is a tyrosine kinase inhibitor (TKI) drug, which is the standard treatment for CML. Nicardipine and amlodipine are calcium channel blockers. Carbamazepine is used to treat seizure disorders; warfarin is an anti-coagulant.

57. The correct answer is (D). Pityriasis rosea is a self-limited skin condition affecting all age groups. The condition can be preceded by a "herald patch." Treatment is supportive.

58. The correct answer is (C). Placental abruption is the separation of the placenta from the uterine wall. Placental abruption usually requires delivery of the fetus. Risk factors for abruption include smoking, hypertension, alcohol abuse, and advanced maternal age.

59. The correct answer is (B). Rheumatoid arthritis is a chronic inflammatory disease in which the immune system affects the joints. The disease is progressive and causes widespread joint destruction. Treatment often consists of NSAIDs, prednisone, and immunosuppressant medications such as methotrexate. Newer medications include Infliximab and Etanercept.

60. The correct answer is (E). Even though it is an invasive tissue, a hydatidiform mole is not malignant. However, if any portion of it is left behind after a procedure such as dilation and curettage, it may lead to the development of a carcinoma. Considering the age of this patient, no risk should be taken; hysterectomy is the best option.

61. The correct answer is (D). *H. pylori* bacterial infection is implicated in the majority of cases of nonerosive chronic gastritis. Chronic erosive gastritis, which involves deterioration of the stomach lining, is most commonly caused by long-term use of non-steroidal anti-inflammatory (NSAID) medications.

62. The correct answer is (B). Acanthosis nigricans is a velvety hyper-pigmented appearance of the skin folds, especially around the neck and axilla. This condition often heralds the presence of insulin resistance. Patients with family history of diabetes and this condition should be closely observed for the onset of diabetes.

63. The correct answer is (A). Mitral valve prolapse is a fairly common heart condition affecting women more often than men. Many patients are asymptomatic; however, some may have symptoms such as palpitations. Maneuvers such as squatting and standing can be used to confirm the diagnosis. Mitral valve prolapse is also known as systolic click-murmur syndrome.

64. The correct answer is (B). This patient is in status epilepticus, which is defined as having more than 30 minutes of continuous seizure activity. Status epilepticus can also be defined as having two or more sequential seizures without full recovery between episodes. This is a life-threatening condition, and a benzodiazepine like valium is the first-line medication for this condition.

65. The correct answer is (D). ACE inhibitors used to treat hypertension often produce a dry cough. This side effect is believed to result from an increase of the vasodilator bradykinin in the body. The breakdown of bradykinin is blocked by the action of ACE inhibitors.

66. The correct answer is (C). Crohn's disease and ulcerative colitis are classified as inflammatory bowel disease. Crohn's is differentiated from ulcerative colitis in that Crohn's usually involves the large and small intestine. Diagnosis is confirmed by colonoscopy. Crohn's is a progressive disease, and treatment is multifactorial. Medications that suppress the immune system are important in treatment, are some of the newer immunosuppressants such as Azathioprine. Surgery is often necessary in order to treat infected bowel and intestinal obstruction.

67. The correct answer is (A). Pelvic inflammatory disease is characterized by infection of the endometrium, fallopian tubes, and ovaries. Infections such as Chlamydia and Gonorrhoeae, if left untreated, ascend through the cervix to cause infection. Treatment consists of antibiotics, avoidance of sexual intercourse until treatment is complete, and treatment of partners.

68. The correct answer is (C). Ribavirin is commonly prescribed for the treatment of chronic hepatitis C in combination with peginterferon alpha-2a. Interferon beta-1b is used to treat multiple sclerosis.

69. The correct answer is (E). The most common etiology of acromegaly is a benign pituitary tumor. The tumor results in hypersecretion of growth hormone.

70. The correct answer is (C). The index of suspicion for myocardial infarction (MI) should be very high in this patient. Patients with diabetes often have vague symptoms of angina as described by nausea and diaphoresis with exertion. Inferior myocardial infarction can cause an increase in parasympathetic tone precipitating hypotension and bradycardia. Changes in leads II, III, and aVF help to exact the location of the MI.

71. The correct answer is (A). Atomoxetine is a selective norepinephrine reuptake inhibitor (SNRI) used in the treatment of ADHD. It is a non-stimulant drug.

72. The correct answer is (D). A cardiac patient who experiences discomfort upon performing any physical activity, even at rest, is most likely experiencing Class IV heart disease, according to the New York Heart Association Functional Classification.

73. The correct answer is (B). Vitamin D deficiency can produce rickets or osteomalacia in children. Vitamin D supplementation can prevent the condition.

74. The correct answer is (A). The history of a headache of sudden onset that is described as "the worst headache of my life" accompanied by neurologic compromise and nuchal rigidity correlates with the diagnosis of subarachnoid hemorrhage. Ruptured berry aneurysm and AV malformation are the most common cause of subarachnoid hemorrhage.

75. The correct answer is (C). The ultrasound is the first line of imaging performed when someone is suspected of having a gallbladder disorder. It is minimally invasive and highly accurate. The combination of lab work and ultrasound is a reliable way of ruling out stones in the common bile duct. If the results of the ultrasound are negative, other imaging modalities can then be explored.

76. The correct answer is (D). Lyme disease is caused by borrelia burgdorferi, a gram-negative spirochete bacteria. The bacteria is most commonly transmitted through tick bites.

77. **The correct answer is (C).** Addison's disease is characterized by hyperpigmentation, muscle weakness, weight loss, and hypotension. The hyperpigmentation of skin is due to the increased levels of corticotropin and melanocyte-stimulating hormone (MSH) that are released from the damaged adrenal cortex.

78. **The correct answer is (B).** This type of injury is commonly caused by a "FOOSH" injury (fall on outstretched hand). Depending on the placement of the fracture, surgery may be required. Avascular necrosis is a serious complication of scaphoid fracture.

79. **The correct answer is (B).** Diabetes insipidus is due to the inability of the kidneys to conserve water. Diabetes insipidus is classified as central or nephrogenic. Central diabetes insipidus is caused by the inability of the neurohypophysis to secrete antidiuretic hormone (ADH). Nephrogenic diabetes insipidus is caused by failure of the kidneys to respond appropriately to ADH. This patient most likely has central diabetes insipidus from a metastatic tumor.

80. **The correct answer is (A).** Migraine headaches are classically described as unilateral and associated with aura and photo-/phonophobia. Headache that interferes with daily activities and is not relieved by OTC analgesics is often treated effectively as migraine. First-line treatment includes triptan medications such as sumatriptan (Imitrex). If headaches are chronic and severe, effective migraine treatment might entail anti-seizure medications such as Topiramate (Topamax) and Divalproate sodium (Depakote). There are many foods and environmental triggers for migraines; these should be avoided.

81. **The correct answer is (A).** Roflumilast is typically prescribed for maintenance treatment of chronic obstructive pulmonary disorder (COPD). It is a PDE4 inhibitor and is also used in the treatment of asthma.

82. **The correct answer is (D).** This is most likely a case of vasovagal syncope. History and physical examination are the most specific and sensitive ways to evaluate for syncope. The EKG is performed to rule out cardiac involvement. The differential diagnosis for syncope is wide and varied and requires a thorough workup.

83. **The correct answer is (E).** Deficiency of thiamine is the main etiology for beriberi. Thiamine is a B-vitamin (vitamin B_1).

84. **The correct answer is (C).** Abdominal aortic aneurysms are more common in the elderly and people with the history of smoking. In patients who are not having symptoms of rupture, diagnosis can be confirmed with abdominal ultrasound. Surgery to repair the aneurysm is generally recommended when the aneurysm measures over 5 cm.

85. **The correct answer is (E).** Aspirin can be administered for prophylaxis of atherothrombosis in patients with diabetes mellitus type 2. Atherothrombosis is a major cause of death in diabetic patients.

86. **The correct answer is (E).** Absence seizures, also known as "petit mal" seizures, are more common in children than adults. During an absence seizure, the patient appears to stare blankly for a short period of time. As with most seizures, there is no memory of it. Ethosuximide and valproic acid are the most commonly used medications for this disorder.

87. **The correct answer is (A).** Duloxetine (Cymbalta) is a serotonin and norepinephrine reuptake inhibitor (SNRI) used in the treatment of depression. Sertraline, fluoxetine, paroxetine, and citalopram are selective serotonin uptake inhibitor (SSRI) antidepressants that increase serotonin levels.

88. **The correct answer is (E).** Beta-blockers are the drug of choice for the treatment of chronic angina. Calcium channel blockers may also be prescribed.

89. **The correct answer is (D).** Vitamin K can reduce the effectiveness of Warfarin (Coumadin), an anti-coagulant. Patients on Warfarin should aim to keep the consumption of vitamin K in their diets at consistent levels.

90. **The correct answer is (A).** Huntington's disease is an inherited disease that causes the destruction of neurons in the basal ganglia and cerebral cortex. This results in an underproduction of acetylcholine (ACh), which results in the exaggerated movements (chorea). Huntington's disease affects the patient's movement, cognitive function, and psychological state. Other symptoms such as dystonia and impaired gait are also typical findings in Huntington's disease.

91. The correct answer is (D). Otitis media is characterized by otalgia, history of URI, and fever. Management of acute otitis media consists of treatment with antibiotics and analgesics. Management of chronic otitis media often requires the placement of tubes in the tympanic membrane (TM).

92. The correct answer is (D). Pancreatic cancer normally goes undiagnosed until advanced stages of the disease. Its symptoms are similar to those of many other digestive diseases. The CMP will indicate if there are any irregularities in the levels of bilirubin. The amylase and trypsinogen evaluate the function of the pancreas. Lastly, the endoscopic ultrasound is highly accurate in diagnosing pancreatic cancer.

93. The correct answer is (C). The hematoma must be removed surgically to relieve pressure on the brain. Traumatic brain injuries such as epidural hematomas are an emergency situation. Epidural hematomas can lead to increased intracranial pressure, anisocoria, and the alteration of consciousness with low Glasgow scores. The typical CT scan findings are the hyper-dense lenticular-shaped image. Surgical evacuation is necessary to treat this condition after completing the ABCs (open airway, breathing, and circulation) of resuscitation.

94. The correct answer is (C). The parathyroid gland controls the regulation of phosphorus and serum calcium. Hyperparathyroidism results in hypercalcemia. Hyperparathyroidism can be caused by a hyper-functioning parathyroid gland (primary hyperthyroidism). Hyperparathyroidism can also be secondary, usually caused by chronic kidney disease. A rare cause of hyperparathyroidism is multiple endocrine neoplasia.

95. The correct answer is (C). Levonorgestrel/ethinyl estradiol is a combined progesterone and estrogen contraceptive. It is used for the prevention of pregnancy.

96. The correct answer is (A). Raynaud's phenomenon involves vasospasms of the fingers and toes. It may rarely affect the ears and nose. It can be either primary or secondary; onset occurs due to emotional stress or exposure to cold.

97. The correct answer is (B). Surgery is the only option for a patient of this age with primary hyperfunction of the parathyroid gland. Fosamax can suppress osteoclast-mediated bone resorption, but it does not treat the hyperactive gland itself, so the levels of parathyroid hormone will remain high. Radioiodine therapy and Levothyroxine target the thyroid, not the parathyroid gland.

98. The correct answer is (A). Before lumbar puncture is performed, the patient must have a CT of the brain to rule out increased intracranial pressure. In the setting of increased intracranial pressure, a lumbar puncture can cause brain herniation.

99. The correct answer is (D). Oral potassium is commonly prescribed for mild or non-emergency hypokalemia. IV potassium is administered in severe or emergency cases.

100. The correct answer is (C). Bacterial conjunctivitis is commonly caused by Staphylococcus aureus, Pseudomonas aeruginosa, Streptococcus pneumonia, and Hemophilus influenza. *Listeria monocytogenes* causes septicemia, meningitis, and encephalitis.

101. The correct answer is (E). HSV-2 is the main etiology for genital herpes. The HSV-1 virus predominantly causes cold sores but can also cause genital herpes.

102. The correct answer is (E). ACE inhibitors are used for the treatment of nephrotic syndrome. NSAIDs such as Naproxen, Meloxicam, Piroxicam, and Ibuprofen are contraindicated due to nephrotoxicity.

103. The correct answer is (B). Mesalamine (5-aminosalicylic acid) is an anti-inflammatory medication. It is used in maintenance treatment of Crohn's disease and ulcerative colitis.

104. The correct answer is (B). This patient is most likely suffering from acute strep pharyngitis. Strep pharyngitis is most common among 5- to 18-year-olds. The illness begins suddenly and acutely. Abdominal pain and vomiting are common associations. The most effective treatment is with amoxicillin. If patient is allergic, erythromycin or azithromycin may be appropriate choices.

105. The correct answer is (C). Schizophrenia is classified as a psychosis and is characterized by deterioration of appearance, hallucinations, delusions, and changes in speech patterns. Onset is typically in the early 20s. Exact cause is unknown, but it is believed to have a genetic link. Treatment consists of anti-psychotic medications such as clozapine and olanzapine.

106. The correct answer is (B). This patient is likely suffering from myasthenia gravis. Myasthenia gravis is an autoimmune disease in which antibodies destroy acetylcholine receptor cites. Episodes of myasthenia gravis are brought on by stress and activity and are usually abated by rest.

107. The correct answer is (B). Cetirizine (Zyrtec) is an over-the-counter antihistamine commonly used to treat allergic rhinitis. Other commonly used antihistamines are loratidine (Claritin) and diphenhydramine (Benadryl).

108. The correct answer is (A). Cystic fibrosis is an autosomal recessive disorder. It is usually diagnosed in infancy. The disease is caused by increased concentrations of sodium and chloride, which create excessively thick mucus in the chest and bowel. Consequently, patients with cystic fibrosis have chronic lung infections and frequent stooling.

109. The correct answer is (D). Obsessive compulsive disorder is a psychiatric disorder marked by obsessions (repetitive consuming thoughts), which are attempted to be relieved by compulsions (ritualistic behavior). Common obsessions are with contamination, resulting in compulsions of ritualistic washing, checking, and hoarding. Obsessive compulsive disorder can be treated with SSRI medication along with cognitive behavior therapy.

110. The correct answer is (B). Hyponatremia refers to an electrolyte imbalance in which serum sodium levels fall to less than 136 mEq/L. Sodium concentrations are reduced relative to water in the body.

111. The correct answer is (B). Bupropion (Wellbutrin) is an antidepressant used in the treatment of depression. It is also approved by FDA as a smoking cessation medication.

112. The correct answer is (B). Tardive dyskinesia is a result of side effects of antipsychotic medications such as thorazine. Tardive dyskinesia is most often irreversible. Considering the severity of the involuntary movements and the permanence of the condition, alternative antipsychotic medications should be strongly considered in most cases of schizophrenia.

113. The correct answer is (C). *Molluscum contagiosum* is caused by the *Molluscum contagiosum* virus (MCV). It is spread through skin-to-skin contact, contact with an inanimate object, and sexual contact.

114. The correct answer is (A). Narcissistic personality disorder is marked by inflated self-esteem and lack of empathy. People with this disorder can often be very charming and engaging but are vulnerable even to the slightest disappointment or criticism. When disappointed, they often become enraged. Because of this behavior, they frequently have problems staying in a regular job and maintaining relationships.

115. The correct answer is (A). Body dysmorphic disorder can be effectively treated by SSRI antidepressants. SGAs are used to treat schizophrenia.

116. The correct answer is (C). Meloxicam is commonly prescribed for treatment of rheumatoid arthritis, osteoarthritis, and juvenile rheumatoid arthritis. It is a nonsteroidal anti-inflammatory drug (NSAID).

117. The correct answer is (D). This patient most likely has secondary hypertension. Lack of family history, early onset, and failure to respond to maximum doses of three BP medications justify a workup for secondary hypertension. Pheochromocytoma is the most likely diagnosis in this patient. Thyroid function tests are also reasonable in order to rule out hyperthyroidism that may cause similar symptoms.

118. The correct answer is (C). Metformin should not be administered to diabetes patients with renal failure, liver failure, or congestive heart failure. Metformin is contraindicated due to the risk of lactic acidosis in patients with these conditions.

119. The correct answer is (B). Tension headaches are the most common form of headaches. They are more common in women than men. They may occur at any age. A headache that has a mild to moderate intensity is most likely a tension headache.

120. The correct answer is (A). Parkinson's disease is a disorder of the basal ganglia and results in decreased dopamine levels. Parkinson's is more common after the age of 60. Parkinson's is also more common in men than women. A resting "pill rolling" tremor is common in Parkinson's. Patients with Parkinson's also have difficulty in initiating movement. Symptoms are commonly experienced unilaterally at onset of the disease.

121. The correct answer is (B). A 65-year old male with microcytic anemia has colon cancer until proven otherwise. Colon cancer occurs most commonly in men and women over the age of 50. Colonoscopy is the most important next test in order to rule out malignancy.

122. The correct answer is (D). Lovastatin is taken to reduce cholesterol. The methotrexate, sulfasalazine, and leflunomide are disease-modifying anti-rheumatic drugs that may be prescribed for rheumatoid arthritis. Rituximab is a biologic anti-neoplastic agent that may also be prescribed.

123. The correct answer is (D). Dextromethorphan is an over-the-counter antitussive commonly used as a cough suppressant. Other common antitussives include codeine and benzonatate.

124. The correct answer is (B). Acyclovir is commonly prescribed for maintenance treatment of genital herpes. It can be taken between outbreaks to prevent or reduce the frequency of their occurrence.

125. The correct answer is (A). This patient has essential or familial tremor. Essential tremor is a benign disorder that is often seen in families. The disorder is worsened by stress and anxiety. It most commonly occurs after the age of 40 but can occur at any age. The patient did not have any other neurological findings, which rules out more malignant neurologic disease.

126. The correct answer is (E). A pterygium is a highly vascularized triangular shaped mass that usually grows from the inner canthus of the eye toward the cornea. It is not to be confused with a pinguccula, which looks like a yellowish fatty deposit on the conjunctiva. Surgical intervention is warranted only when the condition causes a decrease in visual acuity.

127. The correct answer is (D). Fetal alcohol syndrome is a serious result of drinking during pregnancy. The diagnosis of FAS is based on findings of characteristic facial anomalies, growth retardation, and cognitive impairment.

128. The correct answer is (E). Treponema pallidum is the pathogen that causes syphilis. It is best identified through darkfield examination. Because of its small cell diameter, the bacteria is not detected through bright-field microscopy.

129. The correct answer is (E). Albuterol is a short-acting β-2 agonist bronchodilator indicated in the treatment of asthma.

130. The correct answer is (A). Oral candidiasis (thrush) is more common in the very old, the very young, and the immunosuppressed. Hairy leukoplakia can resemble thrush, but it will not scrape off. Treatment includes Mycelex troche or Nystatin oral suspension.

131. The correct answer is (D). ERCP, or endoscopic retrograde cholangiopancreatography, is an invasive procedure used to diagnose and treat conditions of the pancreas. It is a fairly risky procedure that is not heavily used. In addition, this patient is most likely suffering from inflammatory bowel disease, and ERCP would not be appropriate with other signs/symptoms to suggest pancreatitis.

132. The correct answer is (C). Herpes zoster, also known as "shingles," is caused by the reactivation of the chicken pox virus (varicella). The disease appears along a dermatome because of the reactivation of the nerve root. The disease is most common among the elderly and immunosuppressed but can happen in any age group. It affects men and women evenly. Treatment consists of antivirals and analgesics. Antivirals should preferably be used within 72 hours of onset in order to avoid post-herpetic neuralgia (PHN).

133. The correct answer is (D). ACE inhibitors (angiotensin converting enzyme inhibitors) cause vasodilation, thus causing decreased afterload and resulting in easier blood flow through the ventricle. ACE inhibitors are the first line of treatment for patients with left-sided ventricular heart failure and are often used in conjunction with diuretics.

134. **The correct answer is (D).** Chronic thrombocytopenia can be effectively treated with administration of high-dose prednisone. Immunoglobulin may also be prescribed.

135. **The correct answer is (E).** Conversion disorder is commonly treated with psychotherapy. Pharmacologic intervention is not typically indicated; antidepressants may be administered to treat simultaneously occurring depression or anxiety.

136. **The correct answer is (B).** Macular degeneration is caused by the deterioration of the retina. The blind spot in the center of vision is a classic sign of this condition. Macular degeneration is more common in Caucasians in the seventh decade of life. Smoking history, hypertension, and hyperlipidemia are all risk factors for macular degeneration.

137. **The correct answer is (C).** Achalasia is the failure of the lower esophageal sphincter (LES) to relax. Performing an EGD with dilation tears the muscle of the LES to allow food to flow through.

138. **The correct answer is (A).** Meningitis is most likely to occur in winter and spring. The most likely etiology in children is *Neisseria meningitides*. Outbreaks of meningitis are especially common in dormitory situations.

139. **The correct answer is (C).** Hyperthyroidism is primarily caused by Graves' disease. Hyperthyroidism can also be caused by toxic multinodular goiter. Diagnosis is confirmed by suppressed TSH and elevated T3 and T4. First-line treatment is with Tapazole or Propylthiouracil. A beta-blocker such as Inderal can also be used to control palpitations. Surgical intervention and radioiodine therapy should be used when appropriate.

140. **The correct answer is (E).** Spirometry and chest X-ray are important tools both for diagnosing asthma and ruling out other conditions that may cause wheezing. CT scan is not necessary, and peak expiratory flow meters, while helpful in managing asthma, are not helpful in diagnosis.

141. **The correct answer is (C).** Neural tube defects have largely been eradicated through the fortification of grains with folic acid. Other good sources of folic acid are eggs, leafy vegetables such as spinach, and liver. If appropriate amounts of folic acid are not ingested, neural tube defects can occur, usually between the seventeenth and thirtieth days of pregnancy.

142. **The correct answer is (D).** The sweat chloride test is used to diagnose cystic fibrosis. Cystic fibrosis is almost exclusively diagnosed in childhood. A PPD test can help to rule out tuberculosis. A chest X-ray can help rule out a multitude of conditions. A 24-hour pH probe can help to rule out GERD as the cause of chronic cough.

143. **The correct answer is (E).** This patient is exhibiting signs of puberty. Puberty usually begins between the ages of 9 and 14. Earlier development of these symptoms is termed "precocious puberty." The development of these symptoms can cause children to feel alienated from their peers, resulting in depression and acting out.

144. **The correct answer is (A).** This patient most likely has epiglottitis. It is very important NOT to agitate the child. Examination of the pharynx with a tongue depressor can cause airway compromise. The patient should be kept quiet until anesthesia can be administered to secure the airway. Once the patient's airway is secure, more diagnostic tools may be used.

145. **The correct answer is (D).** A Snellen Chart may be used in the evaluation of eye trauma to assess visual acuity. The chart contains letters and/or numbers placed vertically in descending order of size.

146. **The correct answer is (D).** A 65-year old male with microcytic anemia has colon cancer until proven otherwise. Colon cancer occurs most commonly in men and women over the age of 50. The most important risk factor is family history. Studies also show a link to a diet high in animal fat and low in dietary fiber.

147. **The correct answer is (D).** This patient is suffering from atrial fibrillation. All of the other interventions are necessary for rate control and anticoagulation. Anticoagulation is recommended for at least 3 weeks before cardioversion is considered. Immediate cardioversion increases the likelihood of embolic stroke.

148. **The correct answer is (B).** Sildenafil (Viagra) is in a class of medications known as phosphodiesterase-5 (PDE5) inhibitors, commonly used to treat erectile dysfunction. Other PDE5 inhibitors include vardenafil (Levitra) and tadalafil (Cialis).

149. The correct answer is (D). The patient has most likely experienced a transient ischemic attack (TIA). Patients with a history of TIAs are at high risk for strokes. Aspirin prevents the aggregation of platelets and thus clot formation.

150. The correct answer is (D). Malingering is a somatoform psychiatric disorder in which the individual intentionally inflicts or creates symptoms to manifest the appearance of an illness. The goal is typically personal gain, such as in the case of insurance fraud.

151. The correct answer is (A). The patient is most likely suffering from seborrheic dermatitis. The condition is a common condition that usually resolves with the use of OTC shampoos such as Selsun Blue or Ketaconazole. High-potency steroid creams should never be used on the face.

152. The correct answer is (D). Although all of these answer choices can be appropriate in the workup of non-productive cough, the first step is to review the patient's medication list. ACE inhibitors are a common cause of non-productive cough. Some studies show a prevalence of cough in up to 35% of patients treated with the medication.

153. The correct answer is (B). Topical corticosteroids are generally used in combination with antihistamines for the treatment of mild eczema, or atopic dermatitis. Oral corticosteroids such as Prednisolone and Prednisone are used only in severe cases and are not for long-term use.

154. The correct answer is (D). Cushing's disease is caused by excess cortisol hormone. Approximately 60% of cases of Cushing's disease are caused by pituitary microadenomas. ACTH stimulates the adrenal glands to secrete cortisol. Hypersecretion of cortisol is responsible for the characteristic symptoms of Cushing's, such as excess fat between the shoulder blades (buffalo hump), hirsuitism, glucose intolerance, moon facies, and skin changes like acne and telangectasias. Malignancies such as lung cancer can also cause the inappropriate hypersecretion of ACTH. Cushing's disease is just one of the conditions that cause Cushing's syndrome. Causes of Cushing's syndrome include iatrogenic causes, adrenal tumors, and adrenal hyperplasia.

155. The correct answer is (B). The patient's history is consistent with Guillain-Barré syndrome. Guillain-Barré syndrome is marked by ascending paralysis. Causes include, but are not limited to, infections and certain vaccines. In the setting of Guillain-Barré, CSF protein will be increased. EMG determines if the damage is from the nervous system or muscular system. Slowing of the nerve conduction velocity in a nerve conduction study is indicative of Guillain-Barré. Guillain-Barré is associated with Campylobacter jejuni infection.

156. The correct answer is (D). The patient is suffering from a conductive hearing loss as evidenced by the positive Weber's test to the affected ear. Causes of conductive hearing loss include cerumen impaction, otitis media, and otosclerosis. Otosclerosis has the greatest incidence among Caucasian females. Otosclerosis is caused by the abnormal bone formation in the ossicular chain, which conducts sound to the cochlea.

157. The correct answer is (B). Osgood-Schlatter disease refers to osteochondrosis of the tibial tubercle. It involves painful inflammation that worsens with activity.

158. The correct answer is (C). Gemfibrozil is part of the fibrate class of drugs. Fibrates are used to target triglyceride levels specifically. The other options do not focus directly on lowering triglycerides.

159. The correct answer is (C). Prostatitis is an inflammatory condition of the prostate and can be both acute and chronic. Often the symptoms of chronic prostatitis can be vague, consisting of perineal pain, mild dysuria, and/or painful ejaculation. Treatment of chronic prostatitis consists of antibiotics for at least one month.

160. The correct answer is (E). Variant angina is coronary artery spasm that occurs during inactivity, with typical nocturnal onset. It is also known as Prinzmetal's angina.

161. The correct answer is (B). Risperidone is a second-generation antipsychotic (SGA) agent used in the treatment of schizophrenia.

162. The correct answer is (D). The HPV vaccine is administered to prevent infection by the human papillomavirus (HPV). HPV infection is the primary cause of cervical carcinoma and genital warts.

163. **The correct answer is (D).** Clostridium difficile are gram-positive bacilli. Staphylococcus aureus are gram-positive cocci. Bacteroides fragilis and Bordetella pertussis are gram-negative bacilli. Neisseria meningitides are gram-negative cocci.

164. **The correct answer is (B).** The most likely diagnosis in this patient is deep venous thrombosis (DVT). The recent immobilization and smoking history should raise the index of suspicion. Other risk factors for DVT include inherited coagulation disorders, trauma, pregnancy, cancer, and estrogen use.

165. **The correct answer is (B).** The patient is experiencing claudication symptoms most likely caused by peripheral arterial disease (PAD). Cyclobenzaprine is a muscle relaxant and is inappropriate in this patient. Risk factors for peripheral arterial disease include smoking history, diabetes, hypertension, hyperlipidemia, and age over 55. Patients diagnosed with PAD should be considered at high risk for coronary artery disease (CAD).

166. **The correct answer is (B).** Nephrolithiasis is characterized by flank pain and hematuria, which is acute in onset. Diagnosis can be confirmed by spiral CT. Treatment consists primarily of hydration and pain control. The size of the stone determines whether it will pass. Stones <4 mm are likely to pass, while those >6 mm are unlikely to pass.

167. **The correct answer is (D).** Erythema multiforme is a hypersensitivity reaction often associated with infections and certain medications. The syndrome is self-limited. Treatment consists of removing the offending agent, if applicable, and symptomatic treatment.

168. **The correct answer is (D).** The bacteria Rickettsia rickettsii is the most common cause of Rocky Mountain Spotted Fever. *Borrelia burgdorferi* is the bacteria that causes Lyme disease.

169. **The correct answer is (B).** Lopressor is a beta-blocker. Beta-blockers work by blocking the effect of adrenalin on the heart, thus decreasing cardiac output and heart rate. This, in turn, lowers the blood pressure and makes the heart beat more slowly and with less force, reducing the chance of angina pectoris.

170. **The correct answer is (A).** Stenosing tenosynovitis occurs when inflammation causes the tendons of the fingers to thicken, so that they do not slide easily when contracted. It is associated with diseases such as diabetes and arthritis. Anti-inflammatory medications can help; however, there is no specific treatment for the condition.

171. **The correct answer is (B).** Heparin is the drug of choice for the prevention of pulmonary embolism. Heparin is anticoagulant for the prevention of clots; streptokinase is a thrombolytic medication used to dissolve clots in acute cases.

172. **The correct answer is (B).** Diabetes insipidus that occurs during pregnancy is treated by desmopressin acetate as the drug of choice. Desmopressin acetate is a synthetic antidiuretic hormone.

173. **The correct answer is (E).** Diabetic retinopathy, cataracts, glaucoma, and macular degeneration are prevalent causes of adult blindness. Blepharitis can lead to secondary complications, including multiple infections, but is not implicated as a widespread cause of blindness.

174. **The correct answer is (B).** Pyelonephritis is marked by fever and flank pain. Often, there is a history of preceding UTI. Risk factors include abnormalities of the urinary tract, diabetes, and immunocompromise. Pyelonephritis is more likely to occur in elderly patients.

175. **The correct answer is (B).** Atherosclerosis results when the arteries thicken and narrow due to plaque buildup on the arterial walls. It is the most common cause of ischemic heart disease.

176. **The correct answer is (D).** Truncus arteriosus is a congential heart defect that can cause cyanosis. The remaining disorders are noncyanotic congenital defects.

177. **The correct answer is (B).** The patient is experiencing signs and symptoms of Parkinson's disease. Treatment for Parkinson's entails Levodopa often combined with Carbidopa (Sinemet).

178. **The correct answer is (C).** Metoclopramide is commonly prescribed in the treatment of gastroparesis, or delayed gastric emptying. Erythromycin may also be prescribed.

179. The correct answer is (B). The most common causes of dilated cardiomyopathy are post-infarction, valvular heart disease, hypertension, alcoholism, and idiopathic.

180. The correct answer is (C). Dermatophytes are fungi that utilize keratin as a nutrient source. Potassium hydroxide (KOH) preparations are useful for identifying dermatophytes, as the KOH destroys nonfungal cells but not the fungi.

181. The correct answer is (C). Albendazole is commonly used to treat ascariasis resulting from infection by the parasitic roundworm Ascaris lumbricoides. Mebendazole or Ivermectin may also be prescribed. Mild cases of ascariasis typically resolve without treatment.

182. The correct answer is (C). Patients with Still's disease typically display high fever and a characteristic rash. Still's disease is a systemic form of Juvenile Idiopathic Arthritis (JIA).

183. The correct answer is (C). Increased dietary fluids and salt intake can help to counteract mild orthostatic hypotension. Pharmacologic interventions may be indicated in moderate to severe cases.

184. The correct answer is (D). Alzheimer's disease (AD) is the most common form of dementia. It is a progressive, degenerative brain disorder that is characterized by the disturbance of multiple cortical functions. People over the age of 70 are at higher risk for AD. It is also more prevalent in women and African Americans. Rivastigmine is an important part of therapy for patients with Alzheimer's. Rivastigmine is a cholinesterase inhibitor, hence it increases concentration of acetylcholine. Although Rivastigmine slows the progression of Alzheimer's, the disease remains incurable.

185. The correct answer is (B). *Pneumocystis carinnii* pneumonia is an opportunistic infection common in AIDS patients. When HIV patients are not compliant with their treatment regimens, their CD4 counts may drop and make them susceptible to opportunistic infections. X-ray characteristics are often very vague.

186. The correct answer is (A). This patient is most likely suffering from epiglottitis. If epiglottitis is suspected, measurements must be taken to prepare for intubation in order to secure the delicate airway.

Answers (B), (C), and (D) may be valid in the long-term management of this condition but are not appropriate first steps. Answer (E) is inappropriate as attempting to visualize the pharynx with a tongue depressor can both agitate the child and compromise the airway. Epiglottitis is most commonly caused by Haemophilus influenza, and incidence has dropped since introduction of the H. Flu vaccine.

187. The correct answer is (D). Chronic thrombocytopenia can be effectively treated with administration of high-dose prednisone. Immunoglobulin may also be prescribed.

188. The correct answer is (E). Risperidone is a pyschopharmaceutical used in the treatment of schizophrenia. It is in the class of second-generation antipsychotic (SGA) drugs. Individuals undergoing treatment with risperidone are at greater risk for metabolic syndrome, including weight gain and Type 2 diabetes.

189. The correct answer is (E). Damage to the pituitary or hypothalamus through head trauma is a common cause of diabetes insipidus. The decreased specific gravity and osmolality are also key signs of diabetes insipidus. The positive vasopressin challenge test confirms the diagnosis of diabetes insipidus.

190. The correct answer is (A). Barrett's esophagus is an irregular change of the cells that line the esophagus. Photodynamic therapy (PDT) destroys the targeted tissues in hopes of preventing these cells from becoming cancerous.

191. The correct answer is (A). Stable angina is defined as chest pain caused by coronary artery disease that has a predictable pattern. It is common for patients with a cardiac history to complain of chest pain with certain activities. A change in the pattern of angina warrants further investigation.

192. The correct answer is (D). Shigellosis, or dysentery, is not effectively treated by ampicillin, due to increased bacterial resistance. Current treatments include TMP/SMX, ciprofloxacin, or other fluoroquinolone antibiotics such as levofloxacin or norfloxacin.

193. The correct answer is (B). With both bones broken, one bone cannot be used to stabilize the other. Using a cast alone will not guarantee the proper realignment of the arm; both of the bones still have the ability to dislocate. There is also risk of injury to blood vessels and nerves that pass between these bones. Surgery is required to properly secure the bones in place.

194. The correct answer is (C). The most common etiology of otitis externa is Pseudomonas auruginosa. Thorough workup in a patient with diabetes is warranted because of the risk of malignant otitis externa.

195. The correct answer is (E). Cefepime is an important antibiotic in the treatment of osteomyelitis, especially in the treatment of multi-resistant microorganisms such as P. aeruginosa. This organism is resistant to the other options given.

196. The correct answer is (C). Treatment for generalized anxiety disorder generally involves administration of selective serotonin reuptake inhibitors (SSRIs). Haloperidol is an antipsychotic medication.

197. The correct answer is (C). Aside from pancreatitis caused by excessive alcohol consumption, the most common causes of pancreatitis are hypertriglyceridemia, common bile duct stones, lupus, and viral infections such as Hepatitis A. A colonoscopy is the only test that has limited value in diagnosing pancreatitis.

198. The correct answer is (E). Although this patient is a juvenile, Type II diabetes in this age group is rapidly increasing in the United States. Obesity and Hispanic or African American race are risk factors for developing diabetes. Random plasma glucose >200 and signs/symptoms of diabetes warrant the diagnosis of diabetes. Diabetes can also be diagnosed with two separate readings of fasting glucose >126 mg/dL. "Juvenile Diabetes" and "Adult Onset Diabetes" are no longer proper classifications of this disease.

199. The correct answer is (B). This patient is most likely experiencing a pulmonary embolus as evidenced by symptoms and EKG. The next most important test to confirm the diagnosis is a CT of the chest. Other important tests are venous Doppler of the lower extremities and D-Dimer.

200. The correct answer is (B). An EGD is very risky because the patient is exhibiting signs of portal hypertension. A patient in this stage of cirrhosis will have dilation of veins in the esophageal area and low prothrombin levels as well. Performing the EGD procedure could cause perforation of the varicose veins, which could lead to severe bleeding and thus could be lethal for the patient.

201. The correct answer is (C). Chronic obstructive pulmonary disease (COPD) is characterized by chronic cough, wheezing, and dyspnea. The largest risk factor for COPD is smoking. Treatment is centered on smoking cessation. Medications such as inhaled bronchodilators and inhaled steroids are also effective. Oral antibiotics and steroids are often necessary to treat exacerbations of COPD.

202. The correct answer is (B). Acute lymphoblastic leukemia is the most common childhood cancer. Most children on presentation have thrombocytopenia and leukocytosis. Current treatment measures have improved cure rates to 80–90%.

203. The correct answer is (A). A spot urine test uses a sample size of 10–20 mL. Spot urine tests can be conducted to aid in the diagnosis of multiple conditions.

204. The correct answer is (E). Slipped capital femoral epiphysis is a hip disorder that commonly occurs in children ages 11–15, particularly obese children. When adults present with the disorder, endocrine dysfunction such as hypothyroidism should be suspected.

205. The correct answer is (C). This woman most likely contracted viral hepatitis from a blood transfusion. Hepatitis C is a very common cause of hepatitis. Hepatitis B is less likely to cause chronic infection.

206. The answer is (B). Aortic regurgitation can be both congenital and acquired. Acquired causes of aortic regurgitation include endocarditis, aortic aneurysm, and connective tissue disease. Congenital disease is often caused by a bicuspid aortic valve.

207. The correct answer is (E). Naloxone is administered as an antidote in the treatment of opioid overdose, including morphine and heroine. Flumazenil is administered as an antidote in the treament of benzodiazepine overdose.

208. The correct answer is (C). These simple tests done with a tuning fork can help determine the etiology of hearing loss. The Weber test is performed by striking the tuning fork and holding it in the middle of the forehead. In conductive hearing loss, the sound will lateralize to the affected ear. In sensorineural hearing loss, the sound will lateralize to the unaffected ear. The Rinne test is performed by striking a fork and placing it on the mastoid tip. When the patient no longer hears the sound, the fork is placed beside the ear. In conductive hearing loss, the sound will be louder on the mastoid tip than beside the ear (bone conduction > air conduction). In sensorineural hearing loss and in a normal ear, the sound will be louder beside the ear than on the mastoid tip.

209. The answer is (B). Mitral regurgitation is often asymptomatic. Valve abnormalities can be congenital and also acquired. Mitral regurgitation is very common in patients with lupus erythematosus.

210. The correct answer is (B). This patient is most likely suffering from sleep apnea. Physical exam features that suggest sleep apnea are obesity, large neck size, and non-redundant palate. Overnight oximetry can help to confirm the diagnosis of sleep apnea.

211. The correct answer is (C). Acetaminophen is an appropriate treatment for rubella virus, or German Measles. There is no specific treatment for the condition outside of supportive therapy, which may include administration of acetaminophen or ibuprofen.

212. The correct answer is (D). Tourette syndrome is marked by uncontrolled movements and vocal outbursts, known as tics. Tourette affects boys more commonly than girls at a ratio of 3:1. Tics can be varied in nature, but blinking and throat clearing are very common.

213. The correct answer is (A). Arterial flow studies. Peripheral arerial disease (PAD) involves the accumulation of plaque in the arteries. Arterial flow studies are the most useful tool to diagnosis this condition.

214. The correct answer is (D). This patient's smoking history and presentation of unilateral serous otitis media suggests the presence of malignancy. It is important to rule out tumors that might be blocking the Eustachian tube in the nasopharynx, thus inhibiting proper pressure clearance in the middle ear.

215. The correct answer is (C). Lithium is a psychopharmaceutical used in the treatment of bipolar disorder Type 1.

216. The correct answer is (D). Calcium channel blockers are the mainstay treatment for coronary artery spasm (CAS). They operate by slowing the rate at which calcium enters the heart and vessels, thus relaxing the vessels and allowing the blood to flow more freely.

217. The correct answer is (E). A Mallory-Weiss tear is a tear of the mucous membrane of the esophagus. An endoscopy is performed to confirm the diagnosis.

218. The correct answer is (E). Delirium is marked by an acute change in mental status. The most critical step in treating delirium is determining the underlying cause. In this case, the patient was inadequately treated for urinary tract infection. Urinary tract infections are a common cause of delirium in elderly patients.

219. The correct answer is (B). Upper endoscopy is over 95% accurate at diagnosing peptic ulcers. The other tests, while possibly appropriate, are not as specific as upper endoscopy.

220. The correct answer is (C). Cluster headaches are less common than migraine headaches but are similar in nature. The headaches tend to occur in bouts and often at the same time of day. The headaches are often associated with lacrimation, ptosis, and erythema of the conjunctiva on the affected side. Cluster headaches occur most commonly in men.

221. The correct answer is (A). The other diagnostic modalities listed may be appropriate but are not specific tests to identify gouty arthritis. X-ray cannot usually differentiate from other conditions. Uric acid levels can be elevated, but mild kidney disease can also raise levels. A negative rheumatoid factor would rule out rheumatoid arthritis, but a positive test does not rule out gout. An ESR can be elevated in a number of conditions, including all kinds of arthritis.

222. The correct answer is (C). This patient most likely is suffering from an abdominal aortic aneurysm. CT scan will help determine the size of the aneurysm and whether surgery is necessary. It is generally recommended that aneurysms larger than 5 cm be repaired.

223. The correct answer is (C). Fracture of the fifth metacarpal is often called "boxer's fracture," because it commonly occurs during a fight. Treatment is based on severity and may include surgery and/or casting.

224. The correct answer is (D). Phenytoin is a commonly prescribed anticonvulsant used to treat most types of seizure disorders. Side effects are more likely with prolonged use of the medication. Cerebellar ataxia and gingival hyperplasia are two of the most common side effects of phenytoin.

225. The correct answer is (B). People with bipolar disorder are frequently misdiagnosed with depression because they tend to present during periods of depression. Specific questioning about "highs and lows" is important in order to rule out bipolar disorder. Anti-depressants, such as SSRI medications, can sometimes trigger these "manic episodes" because they are energizing.

226. The correct answer is (C). The most likely diagnosis in this scenario is an ectopic pregnancy. Beta hCG and pelvic ultrasound will help to confirm this diagnosis. Pelvic inflammatory disease is also on the differential, hence GC/chlamydia tests are not altogether inappropriate.

227. The correct answer is (B). Any time oxygen will be used for a prolonged period of time, a humidifier should be put in place. Attaching a humidifier to the oxygen tank will to help prevent nasal dryness and irritation of the respiratory tract.

228. The correct answer is (D). Chronic thrombocytopenia can be effectively treated with administration of high-dose prednisone. Immunoglobulin may also be prescribed.

229. The correct answer is (A). Patients with a family history of sudden cardiac death and unexplained syncope should be examined for Long QT syndrome. This disorder can be both congenital and acquired. Certain medications, including quinolone antibiotics, can cause Long QT syndrome.

230. The correct answer is (C). Empyema is a pleural effusion involving the accumulation of pus in the pleural space. Mainstay treatment involves removal of pus from the pleural cavity and administration of antibiotics. Penicillin is commonly prescribed.

231. The correct answer is (A). Streptococcus pneumoniae is the most common cause of pneumonia. Gram's stain of sputum if available would help to establish the diagnosis. Chest X-ray showing consolidation would also be a helpful tool.

232. The correct answer is (D). Most low back pain complaints can be diagnosed with a history and physical. Imaging techniques are indicated when there are "red flags" for more serious conditions, such as motor weakness, bowel/bladder dysfunction, constitutional symptoms, night pain, or immunosuppression.

233. The correct answer is (D). Giardiasis is commonly treated by the anti-parasitic drug Metronidazole. Quinine is an anti-malarial drug; Lindane is used against scabies; and Miconazole is an anti-fungal agent.

234. The correct answer is (B). This patient is suffering from nasal polyps. Patients with nasal polyps often have the triad of asthma, nasal polyps, and aspirin allergy.

235. The answer is (B). Tricuspid regurgitation does not always cause symptoms. This patient most likely had infective endocarditis due to IV drug use, which caused the destruction of the tricuspid valve.

236. The correct answer is (D). All of the diagnostic tools are important in confirming the diagnosis of an ACL tear except for arthrocentesis. The patient has both a history of injury and symptoms of a tear. Arthrocentesis would be helpful in the diagnosis of gout or joint infection.

237. The correct answer is (A). Allergic rhinitis usually occurs with certain seasons (fall and spring), but it can occur throughout the year, depending on the population and climate. The symptoms of sinusitis and rhinitis can be very similar, but the sneezing and watery eyes are what distinguish this patient's condition from sinusitis.

238. The correct answer is (D). Concussions are very common after motor vehicle accidents. Treatment includes careful observation and abstaining from vigorous activities that might cause further injury.

239. The correct answer is (E). Intraosseous administration is superior to intramuscular administration and analogous to intravenous administration. With intraosseous administration, the medication is administered directly into the bone marrow, thus feeding directly into the systemic venous system.

240. The correct answer is (C). Multiple sclerosis is marked by degeneration of the myelin sheath. Patients with preexisting autoimmune diseases such as hypothyroidism are at higher risk for this disease. Females are twice as likely as males to develop this disease, and the onset is normally between the ages of 20 and 40. Patients of Northern European descent are at the highest risk for MS. Lhermitte's sign, which is the feeling of an electrical shock originating in the neck, is a classic symptom in patients with multiple sclerosis. Oligoclonal bands in the CSF also help to confirm the diagnosis of MS.

APPENDICES

Disorders Tested on the PANRE

1. CARDIOVASCULAR DISORDERS

- Cardiomyopathy
- Conduction disorders
- Congenital heart disease
- Heart failure
- Hypertension
- Hypotension
- Coronary heart disease
- Vascular disease
- Valvular disease

2. DERMATOLOGICAL DISORDERS

- Acneiform lesions
- Bacterial infections
- Desquamation
- Eczematous eruptions
- Fungal infections
- Hair conditions
- Insect-related disorders
- Nail conditions
- Neoplasms
- Papulosquamous diseases
- Parasitic disorders
- Verrucous lesions
- Vesicular bullae
- Viral diseases

3. EYE, EARS, NOSE, AND THROAT (EENT) DISORDERS

- Candidiasis
- Cataracts
- Conjunctivitis
- Corneal ulcers or abrasions
- Eustachian tube dysfunction
- Foreign bodies in the eye, ear, nose, or throat
- Gum disease
- Hearing impairment
- Herpes simplex
- Laryngitis
- Macular degeneration
- Mastoiditis
- Ménière's disease
- Otitis media
- Retinal disorders
- Rhinitis
- Sinusitis
- Tinnitus
- Vertigo

4. ENDOCRINE DISORDERS

- Diabetes mellitus
- Hypercholesterolemia
- Hyperparathyroidism
- Hyperthyroidism
- Hypertriglyceridemia
- Hypoparathyroidism
- Hypothyroidism
- Lipid disorders
- Thyroiditis

5. GASTROINTESTINAL DISORDERS

- Appendicitis
- Celiac disease
- Constipation
- Diarrhea
- Esophageal disorders
- Gallbladder disease
- Gastritis
- Hepatitis
- Hernias
- Inflammatory bowel disease
- Irritable bowel syndrome
- Metabolic disorders
- Nutritional deficiencies
- Pancreatic disorders
- Rectal disorders
- Reflux disease
- Vitamin deficiencies

6. GENITOURINARY DISORDERS

- Bladder carcinoma
- Chronic kidney disease
- Cystitis
- Erectile dysfunction
- Incontinence
- Nephrotic syndrome
- Polycystic kidney disease
- Prostate carcinoma
- Prostatitis
- Renal cell carcinoma
- Renal failure
- Renal vascular disease
- Testicular carcinoma
- Urethritis

7. HEMATOLOGIC DISORDERS

- Coagulation disorders
- Hemolytic anemia
- Iron deficiency
- Leukemias, acute and chronic
- Lymphoma
- Multiple myeloma
- Sickle cell anemia

8. INFECTIOUS DISEASES

- Botulism
- Candidiasis
- Chlamydia
- Cholera
- Cryptococcosis
- Diphtheria
- Herpes simplex
- HIV
- Human papillomavirus infections
- Influenza
- Lyme disease
- Malaria
- Measles
- Mumps
- Pinworms
- Rubella
- Shigellosis
- Syphilis
- Tetanus
- Toxoplasmosis
- Tuberculosis

9. MUSCULOSKELETAL DISORDERS

- Back strain/sprain
- Fibromyalgia
- Fractures/dislocations
- Ganglion cysts
- Gout
- Kyphosis
- Low back pain
- Osteoarthritis
- Osteomyelitis
- Osteoporosis
- Reiter syndrome
- Rheumatoid arthritis
- Scleroderma
- Scoliosis
- Soft tissue injuries
- Spinal stenosis

10. NEUROLOGIC DISORDERS

- Cerebral aneurysm
- Cerebral palsy
- Concussion
- Delirium
- Dementias
- Encephalitis
- Headaches
- Huntington's disease
- Meningitis
- Multiple sclerosis
- Parkinson's disease
- Peripheral neuropathies
- Seizure disorders
- Stroke

- Syncope
- Tourette syndrome
- Transient ischemic attack

11. PSYCHIATRIC DISORDERS

- Anorexia nervosa
- Attention deficit/hyperactivity disorder
- Autistic disorder
- Bipolar disorder
- Borderline personality disorder
- Bulimia nervosa
- Conduct disorders
- Depressive disorder
- Domestic violence
- Generalized anxiety disorder
- Grief reaction
- Obesity
- Panic disorder
- Phobias
- Post-traumatic stress disorder
- Schizophrenia
- Substance abuse

12. PULMONARY DISORDERS

- Acute bronchiolitis
- Acute bronchitis
- Acute epiglottitis
- Asthma
- Chronic bronchitis
- Croup
- Cystic fibrosis
- Emphysema
- Influenza

- Lung cancer
- Pertussis
- Pneumonias
- Pulmonary embolism
- Pulmonary hypertension
- Pulmonary nodules
- Sarcoidosis
- Tuberculosis

13. REPRODUCTIVE DISORDERS

- Amenorrhea
- Breast abscess
- Breast carcinoma
- Cervical carcinoma
- Cervical dysplasia
- Cesarean section
- Dysmenorrhea
- Ectopic pregnancy
- Endometrial cancer
- Endometriosis
- Fetal distress
- Galactorrhea
- Gestational diabetes
- Infertility
- Mastitis
- Menopause
- Ovarian cysts
- Ovarian neoplasms
- Pelvic inflammatory disease
- Premenstrual syndrome
- Uterine prolapse
- Vaginal prolapse
- Vaginitis

Organ System List (Details)

1. CARDIOVASCULAR

Circulatory system: Transports nutrients and gases to cells and tissues throughout the body.

Heart

- Pericardium
  - Epicardium
- Myocardium
- Endocardium
- Pulmonary Heart
  - Chordae Tendineae
  - Papillary Muscle
  - Pulmonary Arteries
  - Pulmonary Semilunar Valve
  - Right Atrium
  - Right Ventricle
  - Tricuspid Valve
  - Venae Cavae
- Systemic Heart
  - Aorta
  - Aortic Semilunar Valve
  - Bicuspid Valve
  - Left Atrium
  - Left Ventricle
  - Papillary Muscle
- Conduction System
  - Atrioventricular (AV) Node
  - Sinoatrial (SA) Node
  - Bundle of His
  - Purkinje Fibers

- Coronary Circulation
    - Superior Vena Cava
    - Inferior Vena Cava
    - Aorta
    - Right Coronary Artery
    - Right Marginal Artery
    - Posterior Descending Interventricular Artery
        - Anastomosis
    - Left Anterior Interventricular Artery
    - Left Marginal Artery
    - Left Circumflex Artery
        - Anastomosis
    - Left Coronary Artery
    - Pulmonary Trunk
    - Great Cardiac Vein
    - Middle Cardiac Vein
    - Coronary Sinus
    - Small Cardiac Vein
    - Anterior Cardiac Veins

Blood Vessels of the Body

- Structure of Arteries
    - Tunica Adventitia
    - Tunica Media
    - Tunica Intima
- Structure of Veins
    - Tunica Adventitia
    - Tunica Media
    - Tunica Intima
    - Valves
- Arteries
    - Aorta
    - Systemic Arteries

- Veins
  - Deep Veins
  - Superficial Veins
  - Systemic Veins
- Capillaries
  - Continuous
  - Fenestrated
  - Sinusoidal

Lymph

Lymphatic system: A system of vessels containing lymph, which is a fluid that contains lymphocytes for assisting with immune response. The system also helps to drain interstitial fluid and transport dietary fats, including lipids and fat-soluble vitamins.

Lymphatic System

- Lymph Nodes
- Lymph Vessels
- Tonsils
- Spleen
  - Capsule
  - Red Pulp
  - White Pulp
- Thymus

2. HEMATOLOGIC

Circulatory system: Transports nutrients and gases to cells and tissues throughout the body

Components of Blood

- Erythrocytes (RBC)
  - Blood Groups
    - A
    - B
    - AB
    - O

- o Rhesus Factor
  - • Rh+
  - • Rh–
- Leukocytes (WBC)
  - o Granular
    - • Basophil
    - • Eosinophil
    - • Neutrophil
  - o Agranulocytes
    - • Lymphocytes
      - o B Lymphocytes
      - o T Lymphocytes
      - o Memory Cells
      - o Plasma Cells
    - • Monocytes
      - o Macrophages
- Plasma
  - o Electrolytes
  - o Non-protein Nitrogenous Substances
  - o Nutrients
    - • Carbohydrates
    - • Proteins
    - • Hormones
  - o Proteins
    - • Albumin
    - • Antibacterial Proteins
    - • Globulins (α, β, γ)
    - • Hormones
    - • Metabolic Enzymes
    - • Clotting Proteins
  - o Respiratory Gases
    - • Oxygen
    - • Carbon Dioxide

- Nitrogen
  - Water
- Thrombocytes (Platelets)

Reticuloendothelial System

- Spleen
  - Red Pulp
  - White Pulp
- Bone Marrow
  - Red Marrow
  - Stroma
    - Adipocytes
    - Endothelial Cells
    - Fibroblasts
    - Macrophages
    - Osteoblasts
    - Osteoclasts
  - Yellow Marrow
- Liver

3. DERMATOLOGIC

Integumentary system: Protects the internal structures of the body from damage, prevents dehydration, stores fat, and produces vitamins and hormones.

Skin

- Epidermis
  - Basal Layer
  - Krause Bulbs
  - Ruffini Corpuscles
  - Keratinocytes
  - Melanocytes
  - Langerhans Cells
  - Merkel Cells
  - Meissner Corpuscles
  - Stratum

- Dermis
  - Collagen Bundles
  - Fibroblasts
  - Blood Vessels
  - Lymph Vessels
  - Nerves
  - Pacini Corpuscles
  - Receptors
  - Hair Follicles
  - Sebaceous Glands
  - Sweat Glands
  - Apocrine Glands
  - Skin Derivatives
- Subcutaneous
  - Adipose Tissue
  - Collagen

4. EENT (EARS, EYES, NOSE & THROAT)

Ears

- External Ear
  - Antihelix
  - Antitragus
  - Auricle
  - Concha
  - External Auditory Canal (Ear canal, external auditory meatus, or external acoustic meatus)
  - Fossa Triangularis
  - Helix
  - Intertragic Notch
  - Lobule
  - Scapha
  - Tragus
- Middle Ear
  - Auditory Canal (Eustation)

- ○ Epitympanic Recess
- ○ Eustachian Tube
- ○ Ossicles
  - • Incus
  - • Malleus
  - • Stapes
- ○ Oval Window
- ○ Round Window
- ○ Tensor Tympani
- ○ Tympanic Cavity
- ○ Tympanic Membrane
- • Internal Ear
  - ○ Bony Labyrinth
    - • Cochlea
    - • Semicircular Canals
  - ○ Membranous Labyrinth
    - • Cochlear Nerve
    - • Otoliths
    - • Saccule
    - • Utricle
    - • Vestibular Nerve
    - • Vestibule

Eyes

- • Tunica Fibrosa Oculi
  - ○ Cornea
  - ○ Sclera
- • Lens
  - ○ Lens Capsules
  - ○ Lens Epithelium
  - ○ Lens Fibers
  - ○ Suspensory Ligament
- • Conjunctiva

- - Fornix Conjunctiva
  - Ocular Conjunctiva
  - Palpebral Conjunctiva
- Tunica Vasculosa Oculi
  - Blood Vessels
  - Choroid
  - Ciliary Body
  - Iris
  - Pupil
- Tunica Nervosa Oculi
  - Fovea Centralis
  - Fundus
  - Macula Lutea
  - Optic Disc
  - Retina
    - Amacrine Cells
    - Bipolar Cells
    - Cones
    - Ganglion Cells
    - Horizontal Cell
    - Rods
- Aqueous Humor
- Extraocular Muscles
- Optic Nerve
- Schlemm's Canal
- Vitreous Humor
- Hyaloid Canal

Nose

- External Nose
  - Accessory Nasal Cartilage
  - Ala of Nose (Surface)
  - Greater Alar Cartilage

- - Lateral Nasal Cartilage
  - Lesser Alar Cartilage
  - Nasal Bone
  - Septum Cartilage
  - Vomeronasal Cartilage
- Nasal Cavity
  - Agger Nasi
  - Ethmoid Bulla
  - Ethmoidal Infundibulum
  - Maxilla Hiatus
  - Nasal Conchae
    - Inferior
    - Middle
    - Superior
  - Nasal Meatus
    - Inferior
    - Superior
    - Middle
  - Nasal Septum
  - Nasal Vestibule
  - Nostril
  - Olfactory Mucosa
  - Posterior Nasal Apertures
  - Semilunar Hiatus
  - Sphenoethmoidal recess
  - Vomeronasal Organ
- Paranasal Sinuses
  - Ethmoid
  - Frontal
  - Maxillary
  - Sphenoid
- Olfactory Gland
- Olfactory Bulb
- Cribriform Plate

Throat

- Pharynx
  - Nasopharynx
    - Adenoids
    - Choanae
    - Internal Nares
    - Pharyngeal Opening of Auditory Tube (Eustation)
    - Pharyngeal Recess
    - Torus Tubarius
  - Oropharynx
    - Epiglottic Vallecula
    - Epiglottis
    - Glottis
    - Isthmus Faucium
    - Mouth
    - Palatine Tonsil
    - Palatoglossal Arch
    - Palatopharyngeal Arch
    - Soft Palate
    - Tongue
    - Uvula
  - Laryngopharynx
    - Postcricoid Area
    - Posterior Pharyngeal Wall
    - Pyriform Sinus
- Esophagus
- Hyoid Bone
- Larynx
  - Vocal Folds (Vocal Cords)
  - Vestibular Fold (False Vocal Cords)

5. ENDOCRINE

Endocrine system: Helps to maintain growth and homeostasis within the body through glands that excrete hormones into tissue and blood in the body.

Adrenal

- Cortex
  - Zona Fasciculata
  - Zona Glomerulosa
  - Zona Reticularis
- Medulla
  - Chromaffin Cells

Alimentary System

- Duodenum
  - I Cells
  - S Cells
- Kidney
  - Extraglomerular Mesangial Cells
  - Juxtaglomerular Cells
- Liver
  - IGF
- Pancreas
  - Islets of Langerhans
    - Alpha Cell
    - Beta Cell
    - Delta Cell (D Cells)
    - PP Cell
- Stomach
  - Delta Cells (D Cells)
  - G Cells
  - ECL Cells
  - P/D1 Cells
  - X Cells

Heart

- Cardiac Myocytes

Hypothalamus

- Arcuate Nucleus
  - Dopamine Neurons
  - Neuroendocrine Neurons
- Paraventricular Nucleus
  - Magnocellular Neurosecretory Neurons
  - Neuroendocrine Neurons
- Periventricular Nucleus
  - Parvocellular Neurosecretory Neurons
  - Neuroendocrine Neurons
- Supraoptic Nucleus
  - Magnocellular Neurosecretory Neurons

Ovaries

- Granulosa Cells
- Theca Cells

Parathyroid

- Parathyroid Chief Cell

Pineal Gland

- Pinealocytes

Pituitary Gland

- Adenohypophysis (Anterior Pituitary)
  - Corticotrophs
  - Gonadotrophs
  - Lactotrophs
  - Melanotrophs
  - Somatotrophs
  - Thyrotrophs
- Neurohypophysis (Posterior Pituitary)

- ○ Magnocellular Neurosecretory Cells
- ○ Parvocellular Neurosecretory Neurons

Placenta

- Fetal Trophoblasts
- Syncytiotrophoblast

Skin

- Epidermis
  - ○ Stratum corneum
  - ○ Stratum lucidum (palms of hand and soles of feet)
  - ○ Stratum granulosum
  - ○ Stratum spinosum
  - ○ Stratum germinativum (or stratum basale)
- Basement Membrane
- Dermis
- Papillary Region
- Reticular Region
- Hypodermis

Testis

- Leydig Cells
- Sertoli Cells

Thymus

- Medulla
- Cortex

Thyroid

- Parafollicular Cells
- Thyroid Epithelial Cells

Uterus

- Decidual Cells

6. GASTROINTESTINAL/NUTRITIONAL

Digestive system: Breaks down food polymers into smaller molecules to provide energy for the body.

Alimentary Canal

- Mouth
  - Gingiva
  - Salivary Glands
    - Mucous Tubule
    - Myoepithelial Cell
    - Parotid
    - Salivary Duct
    - Serous Acinus
    - Sublingual
    - Submandibular
  - Soft Palate
    - Palatine Tonsil
    - Palatoglossal Arch
    - Palatopharyngeal Arch
    - Uvula
  - Teeth
    - Alveolar Bone
    - Artery
    - Cementum
    - Dentin
    - Enamel
    - Gingiva
    - Nerve
    - Peridontal Ligament
    - Pulp
    - Pulp Cavity
    - Root Canal
    - Vein
  - Tongue
    - Filiform Papillae
    - Foliate Papillae

- Fungiform Papillae
- Lingual Tonsil
- Vallate Papillae
- Pharynx
  - Nasopharynx
    - Adenoids
    - Choanae
    - Internal Nares
    - Pharyngeal Opening of Auditory Tube (Eustation)
    - Pharyngeal Recess
    - Torus Tubarius
  - Oropharynx
    - Epiglottic Vallecula
    - Epiglottis
    - Glottis
    - Isthmus Faucium
    - Mouth
    - Palatine Tonsil
    - Palatoglossal Arch
    - Palatopharyngeal Arch
    - Soft Palate
    - Tongue
    - Uvula
  - Laryngopharynx
    - Postcricoid Area
    - Posterior Pharyngeal Wall
    - Pyriform Sinus
- Esophagus
  - Lower Esophageal Sphincter (LES)
  - Upper Esophageal Sphincter (UES)
- Peritoneum
  - Common Mesentery
  - Greater Sac

- o Omental Bursa
  - • Greater Omentum
  - • Lesser Omentum
- o Parietal Peritoneum
  - • Peritoneal Cavity
- o Sigmoid Mesocolon
- o Transverse Mesocolon
- o Visceral Peritoneum
- o Falciform Ligament
- Stomach
  - o Body
  - o Cardia
  - o Fundus
  - o Pylorus
- Small intestines
  - o Duodenum
    - • Ascending
    - • Descending
    - • Horizontal
    - • Superior
  - o Ileum
  - o Jejunum
- Large intestines
  - o Anus
  - o Ascending Colon
    - • Ileocecal Valve (ICV)
  - o Cecum
    - • Vermiform Appendix
  - o Descending Colon
  - o Omental Appendices
  - o Rectum
  - o Sigmoid Colon
  - o Taenia Coli

      ○ Transverse Colon

Liver

- Glisson's Capsule
- Caudate Lobe
- Coronary Ligament
- Falciform Ligament
- Hilum
- Left Lobe
- Ligamentum Teres
- Ligamentum Venosum
- Liver Capsule
- Liver Sinusoid
- Quadrate Lobe
- Right Lobe
- Transverse Fissure
- Triad
- Triangular Ligament

Hepatic Biliary System

- Bile Canaliculi
- Canals of Hering
- Interlobular Bile Ducts
- Left Hepatic Duct
- Right Hepatic Duct
- Bile Ductules
  - ○ Anastomosis
- Common Bile Duct
- Sphincter of Oddi

Hepatic Circulation

- Hepatic Artery
- Hepatic Portal Vein
- Central Vein
- Sinusoids

- Hepatic Veins
- Tributary of Hepatic Vein
- Vena Cava

Gallbladder

- Body
- Fundus
- Neck

Gallbladder Biliary System

- Cystic Duct
- Common Bile Duct
- Hepatopancreatic Ampulla
    - Sphincter of Ampulla

Pancreas

- Tail
- Body
- Neck
- Head
    - Uncinate Process

Pancreatic Biliary System

- Common Bile Duct
- Sphincter of Oddi
- Pancreatic Duct
- Hepatoduodenal Ampulla
- Interlobular Duct
- Accessory Pancreatic Duct
    - Minor Duodenal Papilla

Pancreatic Circulation

- Celiac Artery
- Gastroduodenal Artery
    - Superior Pancreaticoduodenal Artery
        - Anterior

- Posterior
- Superior Mesenteric Artery
  - Inferior Pancreaticoduodenal Artery
    - Anterior
    - Posterior
    - Splenic Artery
  - Anastomoses
- Arteria Pancreatica Magna
- Splenic Vein
- Superior Mesenteric Vein
- Portal Vein

7. GENITOURINARY

Urinary/Excretory systems: Remove waste and maintain water balance in the body.

Kidneys

- Renal Fascia
- Renal Capsule
- Renal Cortex
  - Renal Column
- Renal Hilum
- Renal Lobe
- Renal Medulla
  - Renal Sinus
  - Renal Papilla
  - Medullary Interstitium
  - Renal Pyramids
- Cortical Lobule
- Medullary Ray
- Nephron
- Renal Tubule
  - Renal Corpuscle
    - Glomerulus
    - Bowman's Capsule

- ○ Proximal Tubule
- ○ Loop of Henle
  - • Descending
  - • Thin Ascending
  - • Thick Ascending
- ○ Distal Convoluted Tubule
- ○ Connected Tubule
- ○ Collecting Ducts
- ○ Renal Papilla
- ○ Minor Calyx
- ○ Major Calyx
- ○ Renal Pelvis
- • Juxtaglomerular Apparatus
  - ○ Macula Densa
  - ○ Juxtaglomerular Cells
  - ○ Mesangium
  - ○ Extraglomerular Mesangial Cell
- • Filtration
  - ○ Glomerular Basement Membrane
  - ○ Podocyte
  - ○ Filtration slits
  - ○ Intraglomerular Mesangial Cell
  - ○ Tubular Fluid

Renal Circulation

- • Intrarenal Arteries
  - ○ Renal Artery
  - ○ Segmental Arteries
  - ○ Interlobar Arteries
  - ○ Arcuate Arteries
  - ○ Interlobular Arteries
  - ○ Afferent Arterioles
- • Intrarenal Veins
  - ○ Efferent Arterioles

- ○ Peritubular Capillaries
- ○ Vasa Recta
- ○ Arcuate Vein
- ○ Interlobar Veins
- ○ Renal Vein

Ureters

- Pelviureteric Junction
- Ureterovesical Valve
- Orifice of Ureter
- Adventitia
- Muscular Layer
- Mucosa

Urinary Bladder

- Apex
- Uvula
- Neck
- Medial Umbilical Ligament
- Muscular Layer
  - ○ Detrusor Muscle
  - ○ Trigone
- Mucosa
- Submucosa
- Internal Urinary Sphincter
- Ureteral Orifice

Urethra

- Female
  - ○ Membranous Urethra
  - ○ External Urethral Sphincter
- Male
  - ○ Pre-Prostatic Urethra
  - ○ Prostatic Urethra
  - ○ Spongy Urethra

○   External Urethral Sphincter

8. INFECTIOUS DISEASES

Infectious disease: The presence of a microscopic pathological organism that has infected the host, such as bacteria, parasites, viruses, or fungi.

- *Acinetobacter baumannii* Infection
- Acquired Immunodeficiency Syndrome (AIDS)
- Actinomycosis
- Amebiasis (*Entamoeba histolytica*)
- American Trypanosomiasis (Chagas Disease)
- Anthrax
- *Arcanobacterium haemolyticum* Infection
- Argentine Hemorrhagic Fever (AHF)
- Ascariasis (Ascaris lumbricoides)
- Aspergillosis
- Astrovirus Infection
- Babesiosis
- *Bacillus cereus* Infection
- Bacterial Meningitis
- Bacterial Pneumonia
- Bacterial Vaginosis (BV)
- *Bacteroides fragilis* Infection
- Balantidiasis (*Balantidium coli*)
- *Baylisascaris* Infection
- BK Virus Infection
- Black Piedra (Piedraia hortae)
- Blastocystis Infection
- Blastomycosis (Gilchrist's Disease)
- Bolivian Hemorrhagic Fever (BHF)
- *Borrelia burgdorferi* Infection (Lyme Disease)
- Botulism (Botulinum Intoxication)
- Bovine Spongiform Encephalopathy (BSE, Mad-Cow Disease)
- Brazilian Hemorrhagic Fever (BzHF)

- Brucellosis (Bang's Disease, Crimean Fever)
- *Burkholderia cepacia* Complex (BCC)
- Buruli Ulcer (Bairnsdale Ulcer, Searls Ulcer)
- Campylobacteriosis
- Candidiasis (Thrush)
- Cat Scratch Disease (CSD, Cat Scratch Fever)
- Cellulitis
- Chancroid (Soft Chancre)
- Chlamydia Infection
- *Chlamydophila pneumoniae* Infection (TWAR)
- Cholera (*Vibrio cholerae*)
- Chromoblastomycosis (Verrucous Dermatitis)
- Clonorchiasis
- Clostridial Myonecrosis (Gas Gangrene)
- *Clostridium difficile* Infection (Pseudomembranous Colitis)
- Coccidioidomycosis (Valley Fever)
- Colorado Tick Fever (CTF)
- Creutzfeldt-Jakob Disease (CJD)
- Crimean-Congo Hemorrhagic Fever (CCHF)
- Cryptococcosis
- Cryptosporidiosis (Crypto)
- Cutaneous Larva Migrans (CLM)
- Cyclosporiasis
- Cysticercosis (Pork Tapeworm)
- Dengue Fever (Breakbone Fever)
- Dientamoebiasis (Travelers Diarrhea)
- Diphtheria
- Diphyllobothriasis (Fish Tapeworm)
- Dracunculiasis (Guinea Worm Disease)
- Ebola Hemorrhagic Fever (EHF)
- Echinococcosis (Hydatid Disease)
- Ehrlichiosis
- Enterobiasis (Pinworm)

- Enterococcus Infection
- Enterovirus Infection
- Epidemic Parotitis (Mumps)
- Epidemic Typhus (Camp Fever)
- Erythema Infectiosum (Fifth Disease)
- *Escherichia coli* Infection (*E.coli*)
- Fascioliasis (Liver Rot)
- Fasciolopsiasis
- Fatal Familial Insomnia (FFI)
- Filariasis (Philariasis)
- Food Poisoning
- Free-Living Amoebic Infection (FLA)
- *Fusobacterium necrophorum* Infection (Lemierre's Syndrome)
- Geotrichosis
- Gerstmann-Straussler-Scheinker Syndrome (GSS)
- Giardiasis (Beaver Fever)
- Glanders (Equinia)
- Gnathostomiasis (Larva Migrans Profundus)
- Gonorrhea (The Clap)
- Granuloma inguinale (Donovanosis)
- *Haemophilus influenzae* Infection (Pfeiffer's Bacillus)
- Hand, Foot and Mouth Disease (HFMD)
- Hantavirus Pulmonary Syndrome (HPS)
- *Helicobacter pylori* Infection (H.pylori)
- Hemolytic-Uremic Syndrome (HUS)
- Hemorrhagic Fever with Renal Syndrome (HFRS)
- Hepatitis A (HAV, Hep A)
- Hepatitis B (HBV, Hep B)
- Hepatitis C (HCV, Hep C)
- Hepatitis D (HDV, Hep D)
- Hepatitis E (HEV, Hep E)
- Histoplasmosis (Cave Disease)
- Hookworm Infection

- Human African Trypanosomiasis (Sleeping Sickness)
- Human Bocavirus Infection (HBoV)
- Human Ehrlichiosis Ewingii Infection (*Erlichia ewingii*)
- Human Granulocytic Anaplasmosis (HGA)
- Human Herpes Virus 1 (Cold Sores)
- Human Herpes Virus 2 (Genital Herpes)
- Human Herpes Virus 3 (Varicella-Zoster, Chickenpox, Shingles)
- Human Herpes Virus 4 (Epstein-Barr)
- Human Herpes Virus 5 (Cytomegalovirus)
- Human Herpes Virus 6 (Exanthem Subitum, Roseola Infantum)
- Human Herpes Virus 7 (Roseola)
- Human Herpes Virus 8 (Kaposi's Sarcoma)
- Human Immunodeficiency Virus (HIV)
- Human Metapneumovirus Infection (hMPV)
- Human Monocytotropic Ehrlichiosis (HME)
- Human Papillomavirus Infection (HPV)
- Human Parainfluenza Virus Infection (HPIVs)
- Hymenolepiasis
- Impetigo
- Influenza (Flu)
- Isosporiasis
- Kawasaki Disease (KD)
- Keratitis
- *Kingella kingae* Infection
- Kuru (Laughing Sickness)
- Lassa Fever
- Legionellosis (Legionnaires' Disease, Pontiac Fever)
- Leishmaniasis
- Leprosy (Hansen's Disease)
- Leptospirosis (Weil's Syndrome)
- Listeriosis
- Lymphatic Filariasis (Philariasis)
- Lymphocytic Choriomeningitis (LCM)

- Malaria
- Marburg Hemorrhagic Fever (MARV)
- Measles (Rubeola)
- Melioidosis
- Meningitis
- Meningococcal Disease
- Metagonimiasis
- Methicillin-Resistant *Staphylococcus aureus* Infection (MRSA)
- Microsporidiosis
- *Molluscum contagiosum* Infection (MCV)
- Murine Typhus (Endemic Typhus)
- Mycetoma (Eumycetoma)
- Mycobacterial Infection
- *Mycoplasma pneumoniae* Infection (Walking Pneumonia)
- Myiasis
- Nasopharyngitis (Common Cold)
- Neonatal Conjunctivitis (Ophthalmia Neonatorum)
- Nocardiosis
- Norovirus Infection (Norwalk Agent)
- Onchocerciasis (River Blindness)
- Paracoccidioidomycosis (Brazilian Blastomycosis)
- Paragonimiasis
- Pasteurellosis *Pasteurella multocida* (*P. septica*)
- *Pediculosis Capitis* (Head Lice)
- *Pediculosis Corporis* (Body Lice, Vagabond's Disease)
- *Pediculosis Pubis* (Pubic Lice)
- Pelvic Inflammatory Disease (PID)
- Pertussis (Whooping Cough)
- Plague (Bubonic, Septicemic, Pneumonic)
- Pneumococcal Infection
- Pneumocystis Pneumonia (PCP)
- Pneumonia
- Poliomyelitis (Polio)

- *Prevotella intermedia* Infection
- *Prevotella melaninogenica* Infection
- Primary Amebic Meningoencephalitis (PAM)
- Progressive Multifocal Leukoencephalopathy (PML)
- Psittacosis (Parrot Disease)
- Q fever
- Rabies
- Rocky Mountain Spotted Fever
- Rotavirus
- Rubella (German Measles)
- Salmonellosis
- Sapporo Virus Infection
- Scabies (Seven-Year Itch)
- Scarlet Fever (Scarlatina)
- Schistosomiasis (Snail Fever)
- Sepsis (SIRS)
- Severe Acute Respiratory Syndrome (SARS)
- Shigellosis (Bacillary Dysentery)
- Smallpox (*Variola*)
- Sporotrichosis (Rose Gardener's Disease)
- Staphylococcal Infection
- Streptococcal Infection Group A (GAS)
- Streptococcal Infection Group B (GBS)
- Strongyloidiasis (Roundworm)
- Syphilis
- Taeniasis (Beef Tapeworm, Pork Tapeworm)
- Tetanus (Lockjaw)
- Tinea Barbae (Barber's Itch)
- Tinea Capitis (Scalp Ringworm)
- Tinea Corporis (Body Ringworm)
- Tinea Cruris (Jock Itch)
- Tinea Manuum (Hand Ringworm)
- Tinea Nigra

- Tinea Pedis (Athlete's Foot)

- Tinea Unguium (Onychomycosis)

- Tinea Versicolor (Pityriasis Versicolor)

- Toxocariasis (VLM)

- Toxoplasmosis

- Trachoma (Granular Conjunctivitis)

- Trichinellosis

- Trichomoniasis (Trich)

- Trichuriasis (Whipworm Infection)

- Trypanosomiasis

- Tuberculosis (TB)

- Tularemia (Pahvant Valley Plague)

- Typhoid Fever (Typhoid)

- *Ureaplasma urealyticum* Infection

- Urinary Tract Infections

- Venezuelan Equine Encephalitis (VEE)

- Venezuelan Hemorrhagic Fever (VHF)

- Viral Encephalitis

- Viral Gastroenteritis

- Viral Meningitis

- Viral Pneumonia

- West Nile Virus (WNV)

- White Piedra (Tinea Blanca)

- Yellow Fever (Yellow Jack)

- *Yersinia pseudotuberculosis* Infection

- Yersiniosis

- Zygomycosis

9. MUSCULOSKELETAL

Muscular system: Enables movement of the body.

Muscles

- Microscopic Structure of Muscle

  - Sarcomere

- Muscle Fiber
  - Striated Cardiac
  - Striated Voluntary
  - Smooth
- Macroscopic Structure of Muscle
  - Endomysium
  - Epimysium
  - Fasciculus
  - Perimysium
  - Tendon
  - Fascia
  - Origin and Insertion
  - Organization of Fibers
    - Bipennate
    - Circular
    - Convergent
    - Fusiform
    - Multipennate
    - Parallel
    - Unipennate
- Muscles of the Body
  - Facial
    - Frontalis
    - Orbicularis Oculi
    - Temporalis
    - Zygomaticus
    - Masseter
    - Orbicularis Oris
  - Neck
    - Platysma
    - Sternohyoid
    - Sternocleidomastoid
    - Occipitalis

- Trapezius
  - Shoulder
    - Trapezius
    - Deltoid
    - Infraspinatus
    - Teres Major
    - Rhomboid Major
  - Arm
    - Triceps Brachii
    - Biceps Brachii
    - Brachialis
  - Forearm
    - Pronator Teres
    - Brachioradialis
    - Extensor Carpi Radialis Longus
    - Flexor Carpi Radialis
    - Flexor Carpi Ulnaris
    - Extensor Carpi Ulnaris
    - Palmaris Longus
    - Extensor Digitorum
  - Thorax
    - Pectoralis Minor
    - Pectoralis Major
    - Serratus Anterior
    - Intercostals
  - Back
    - Latissimus Dorsi
  - Abdomen
    - Rectus Abdominis
    - External Oblique
    - Internal Oblique
    - Transversus Abdominis
  - Hip

- - Gluteus Medius
  - Gluteus Maximus
  - Pelvis/Thigh
    - Iliopsoas
    - Pectineus
  - Thigh
    - Tensor Fasciae Latae
    - Sartorius
    - Adductor Longus
    - Adductor Magnus
    - Hamstrings
    - Biceps Femoris
    - Gracilis
    - Rectus Femoris
    - Vastus Lateralis
    - Vastus Medialis
    - Iliotibial Tract
    - Semitendinosus
    - Semimembranosus
  - Leg
    - Fibularis Longus
    - Extensor Digitorum Longus
    - Tibialis Anterior
    - Gastrocnemius
    - Soleus
    - Calcaneal Tendon
- Visceral/Smooth Muscle
  - Arrector Pili (Skin)
  - Blood Vessels
  - Ciliary Muscle (Eye)
  - Gastrointestinal Tract
  - Iris (Eye)
  - Lymphatic Vessels

- ○ Mesangial Cells (Kidney)
- ○ Reproductive Tracts
- ○ Respiratory Tract
- ○ Urinary Bladder
- ○ Uterus

Musculoskeletal Circulation

- Arterioles
- Capillaries
- Venules

Skeletal system: Supports and protects the body while giving it shape and form.

Bones

- Flat
- Irregular
- Long
- Sesamoid
- Short

Simplified Human Skeleton

- Skull
  - ○ Frontal Bone
  - ○ Parietal Bones
  - ○ Temporal Bones
  - ○ Occipital Bone
  - ○ Sphenoid Bone
  - ○ Ethmoid Bone
  - ○ Maxilla
  - ○ Mandible
  - ○ Palatine Bones
  - ○ Zygomatic Bones
  - ○ Nasal Bones
  - ○ Lacrimal Bones
  - ○ Vomer
  - ○ Inferior Nasal Conchae

- Hyoid Bone
- Scapula
- Clavicle
- Sternum
- Ribs
- Vertebrae
  - Cervical (C1-C7)
  - Thoracic (T1-T12)
  - Lumbar (L1-L5)
- Humerus
- Ulna
- Radius
- Carpals
  - Scaphoid Bones
  - Lunate Bones
  - Triquetral Bones
  - Pisiform Bones
  - Trapezium
  - Trapezoid Bones
  - Capitate Bones
  - Hamate Bones
- Metacarpals
- Phalanges (Carpal)
  - Proximal
  - Intermediate
  - Distal
- Pelvis
  - Sacrum
  - Coccyx
  - Hipbone
    - Ilium
    - Ischium
    - Pubis

- Femur
- Patella
- Tibia
- Fibula
- Tarsals
    - Calcaneus
    - Talus
    - Navicular Bones
    - Medial Cuneiform Bones
    - Intermediate Cuneiform Bones
    - Lateral Cuneiform Bones
    - Cuboid Bones
- Metatarsals
- Phalanges (Tarsal)
    - Proximal
    - Intermediate
    - Distal

Joints

- Cartilaginous Joint
- Fibrous Joint
- Synovial Joint
    - Ball and Socket Joint
    - Condyloid Joint
    - Hinge Joint
    - Pivot Joint
    - Planar Joint
    - Saddle Joint

Ligaments

Articular Ligaments

Head and neck

    - Cricothyroid ligament

- o Periodontal ligament
- o Suspensory ligament of the lens
- Thorax
  - o Suspensory ligament of the breast
- Pelvis
  - o Anterior sacroiliac ligament
  - o Posterior sacroiliac ligament
  - o Sacrotuberous ligament
  - o Sacrospinous ligament
  - o Inferior pubic ligament
  - o Superior pubic ligament
  - o Suspensory ligament of the penis
- Wrist
  - o Palmar radiocarpal ligament
  - o Dorsal radiocarpal ligament
  - o Ulnar collateral ligament
  - o Radial collateral ligament
- Knee
  - o Anterior cruciate ligament (ACL)
  - o Lateral collateral ligament (LCL)
  - o Posterior cruciate ligament (PCL)
  - o Medial collateral ligament (MCL)
  - o Cranial cruciate ligament (CrCL) - quadruped equivalent of ACL
  - o Caudal cruciate ligament (CaCL) - quadruped equivalent of PCL
  - o Patellar ligament (ACL)

Peritoneal Ligaments

- Hepatoduodental ligament
- Broad ligament of the uterus

Cartilage

- Elastic Cartilage
- Fibrocartilage
- Hyaline Cartilage

Synovial Membranes

- Synovium
  - Outer layer (subintima)
  - Inner layer (intima)

Intervertebral Discs

- Nucleus pulposus
- Annulus fibrosis

10. NEUROLOGIC SYSTEM

Nervous system: Monitors and coordinates internal organ function and responds to changes in the external environment.

Central Nervous System (CNS)

- Brain
- Cranial Nerves
  - Olfactory (I)
  - Optic (II)
  - Oculomotor (III)
  - Trochlear (IV)
  - Trigeminal (V)
  - Abducens (VI)
  - Facial (VII)
  - Vestibulocochlear (VIII)
  - Glossopharyngeal (IX)
  - Vagus (X)
  - Accessory (XI)
  - Hypoglossal (XII)
- Brain Stem
  - Mesencephalon
    - Cerebral Peduncle
    - Mesencephalic Duct
    - Pretectum
    - Tectum

- ○ Rhombencephalon
    - • Cerebellum
    - • Medulla Oblongata
    - • Metencephalon
    - • Myelencephalon
    - • Pons
- • Prosencephalon
    - ○ Diencephalon
        - • Epithalamus
        - • Hypothalamus
        - • Pineal Gland
        - • Pituitary Gland
        - • Subthalamus
        - • Thalamus
        - • Third Ventricle
    - ○ Telencephalon
        - • Amygdala
        - • Basal Ganglia
        - • Hippocampus
        - • Lateral Ventricles
        - • Neocortex
        - • Rhinencephalon
- • Spinal Cord

Peripheral Nervous System (PNS)

- • Spinal Nerves and Branches
    - ○ Cervical Plexus (C1-C4)
    - ○ Brachial Plexus (C5-T1)
    - ○ Lumbosacral Plexus (L1-C0)
- • Autonomic Nervous System
    - ○ Parasympathetic
        - • Digestive (regulates motility and glandular activity)

- ○ Sympathetic
  - Cardiovascular (assists in regulating heart rate and blood pressure)
  - Endocrine (activates the adrenal medulla)
  - Lymphatic (regulates immune function)
  - Muscles (activates skeletal muscles)
  - Reproductive (regulates erections and ejaculation)
  - Respiratory (regulates respiratory rhythm and depth)
  - Skeletal (bones provide calcium needed for neural function)
  - Skin (regulates sweat glands and blood vessels of skin)
  - Urinary (regulates bladder emptying and renal blood pressure)
- Circulatory System of the Brain
  - ○ Circle of Willis
    - Anterior Communicating Artery
    - Anterior Cerebral Artery
    - Internal Carotid Artery
    - Middle Cerebral Artery
    - Ophthalmic Artery
    - Anterior Choroidal Artery
    - Posterior Communicating Artery
    - Posterior Cerebral Artery
    - Superior Cerebellar Artery
    - Basilar Artery
    - Pontine Arteries
    - Anterior Inferior Cerebellar Artery
    - Vertebral Artery
    - Posterior Inferior Cerebellar Artery
    - Anterior Spinal Artery

11. PSYCHIATRY/BEHAVIORAL

Psychiatry/ Behavioral: These mental disorders include various affective, behavioral, cognitive, and perceptual abnormalities.

- Acute Stress Disorder
- Adjustment Disorder

- Agoraphobia
- Amnesia, Dissociative
- Anorexia Nervosa
- Antisocial Personality Disorder
- Anxiety Disorder
- Avoidant Personality Disorder
- Bipolar Disorder
- Body Dysmorphic Disorder
- Borderline Personality Disorder
- Breathing-Related Sleep Disorder
- Brief Psychotic Disorder
- Bruxism
- Bulimia Nervosa
- Cataplexy
- Circadian Rhythm Sleep Disorder
- Conversion Disorder
- Cyclothymic Disorder
- Delusional Disorder
- Dependent Personality Disorder
- Depersonalization Disorder
- Depressive Disorder
- Dissociative Identity Disorder (DID)
- Dyspareunia
- Dyssomnia NOS
- Dysthymic Disorder
- Eating Disorder
- Exhibitionism
- Female Orgasmic Disorder
- Female Sexual Arousal Disorder
- Fetishism
- Frotteurism
- Fugue, Dissociative
- Gender Identity Disorder

- Generalized Anxiety Disorder
- Histrionic Personality Disorder
- Hypoactive Sexual Desire Disorder
- Hypochondriasis
- Hypopnea Syndrome
- Impotence
- Impulse Control Disorder
- Intermittent Explosive Disorder
- Kleptomania
- Major Depressive Disorder
- Male Erectile Disorder
- Male Orgasmic Disorder
- Mixed Type Sleep Disorder
- Mood Disorder
- Narcissistic Personality Disorder
- Narcolepsy
- Nightmare Disorder
- Nocturia
- Obsessive Compulsive Disorder
- Pain Disorder
- Panic Disorder
- Paranoid Personality Disorder
- Paraphilia
- Parasomnia NOS
- Pathological Gambling
- Pedophilia
- Periodic Limb Movement Disorder
- Personality Disorder NOS
- Phobias
- Posttraumatic Stress Disorder
- Premature Ejaculation
- Primary Hypersomnia
- Primary Insomnia

- Psychotic Disorder
- Pyromania
- Restless Legs Syndrome
- Schizoaffective Disorder
- Schizoid Personality Disorder
- Schizophrenia
- Schizophreniform Disorder
- Sexual Aversion Disorder
- Sexual Disorder
- Sexual Dysfunction
- Sexual Masochism
- Sexual Sadism
- Shared Psychotic Disorder
- Sleep Apnea
- Sleep Disorder
- Sleep Paralysis
- Sleep Terror Disorder
- Sleepwalking Disorder
- Social Phobia
- Somatization Disorder
- Somniphobia
- Specific Phobia
- Substance Abuse
- Substance Dependence
- Transvestic Fetishism
- Trichotillomania
- Vaginismus
- Voyeurism

12. PULMONARY

Respiratory system: Provides the body with oxygen via gas exchange between air from the outside environment and gases in the blood.

Nose

Sinuses

- Ethmoid
- Frontal
- Mastoid
- Maxillary
- Sphenoid

Pharynx

- Nasopharynx
    - Adenoids
    - Choanae
    - Cribriform Plate
    - Internal Nares
    - Pharyngeal Opening of Auditory Tube (Eustation)
    - Pharyngeal Recess
    - Torus Tubarius
- Oropharynx
    - Epiglottic Vallecula
    - Epiglottis
    - Glottis
    - Isthmus Faucium
    - Mouth
    - Palatine Tonsil
    - Palatoglossal Arch
    - Palatopharyngeal Arch
    - Soft Palate
    - Tongue
    - Uvula
- Laryngopharynx
    - Postcricoid Area
    - Posterior Pharyngeal Wall
    - Pyriform Sinus

Larynx

- Arytenoid Cartilage
- Corniculate Cartilage
- Cricoid Cartilage
- Cricothyroid Ligament
- Epiglottic Cartilage
- Epiglottis
- Laryngeal Cavity
- Paired Arytenoid Cartilage
- Paired Corniculate Cartilage
- Paired Cuneiform Cartilage
- Rima Glottis
- Thyrohyoid Membrane
- Thyroid Cartilage
- Vestibular Fold
- Vocal Fold

Trachea

- Cartilaginous Rings
- Trachealis Muscle

Bronchus

- Alveolar Ducts
- Alveolar Sacs
- Bronchopulmonary Segment
- Hyaline Cartilage
- Left Main Bronchus
- Lobar Bronchi
- Primary Bronchioles
- Respiratory Bronchioles
- Right Main Bronchus
- Terminal Bronchioles
- Tertiary Bronchi

Lungs

- Lung Capillaries
- Pleurae
- Upper Lobe
  - Apical
  - Anterior
  - Cardiac Notch (Left Lung)
  - Posterior
- Middle Lobe
  - Lateral
  - Medial
- Lower Lobe
  - Basal Anterior
  - Basal Lateral
  - Basal Posterior
  - Superior

Thoracic Diaphragm

- Body Cavity Connections
  - Sternal
  - Costal
  - Lumbar

Pulmonary Circulation

- Right Ventricle
- Pulmonary Semilunar Valve
- Left Pulmonary Artery
- Right Pulmonary Artery
- Bronchial Arteries
- Capillaries
- Pulmonary Veins
  - Right Inferior Pulmonary
  - Right Superior Pulmonary
  - Left Inferior Pulmonary

- ○ Left Superior Pulmonary
- ○ Superior Vena Cava
- ○ Inferior Vena Cava
- ○ Brachiocephalic
  - • Internal Jugular
  - • Subclavian
  - • Pericardiacophrenic
  - • Vertebral
  - • Supreme
  - • Left Superior Intercostal
  - • Internal Thoracic
- ○ Azygos
  - • Right Superior Intercostal
  - • Bronchial
  - • Intercostal
  - • Posterior Intercostal
  - • Hemiazygos
  - • Accessory Hemiazygos
  - • Superior Phrenic
- • Left Atrium
- • Bicuspid Valve
- • Left Ventricle

13. REPRODUCTIVE

Reproductive system: Enables the production of offspring through sexual reproduction.

Males

- • Bulbourethral Gland
- • Ejaculatory Duct
- • Penis
  - ○ Corpus Cavernosum
    - • Crus of Penis
  - ○ Corpus Spongiosum

- - - Bulb of Penis
    - - Glans of Penis
  - ○ Prepuce
- Prostate Gland
- Scrotum
- Seminal Vesicle
- Testis
  - ○ Ductus Deferens
  - ○ Efferent Duct
  - ○ Epididymis
    - - Head
    - - Body
    - - Tail
  - ○ Rete Testis
  - ○ Seminiferous Tubule
  - ○ Tunica Albuginea
    - - Septum
  - ○ Tunica Vaginalis
  - ○ Tunica Vasculosa Testis
- Urethra
  - ○ Bulbourethral Gland
  - ○ Pre-Prostatic Urethra
  - ○ Prostatic Urethra
  - ○ Spongy Urethra
  - ○ Urethral Sphincter

Females

- Mammary glands
  - ○ Areola
  - ○ Glandular Lobe
    - - Lactiferous Duct
    - - Lactiferous Sinus
  - ○ Nipple
  - ○ Pectoralis Muscle

- Superficial Fascia
- Suspensory Ligament
- Ovaries
  - Cortex
  - Follicles
  - Germinal Epithelium
  - Hilus
  - Medulla
  - Stroma
  - Tunica Albuginea
- Oviducts
  - Ampulla
  - Fimbriae
  - Infundibulum
  - Isthmus
  - Tubal Ostium
- Uterus
  - Body
    - Fundus
    - Uterine Cavity
  - Broad Ligament
  - Cardinal Ligament
  - Cervix
  - Endometrium
  - Myometrium
  - Ovarian Ligament
  - Parametrium
  - Perimetrium
  - Pubocervical Ligament
  - Round Ligament
  - Uterine Horns
  - Uterosacral Ligament
- Vagina

- Fornix of Vagina
- Hymen
- Fossa of Vestibule

- Vulva
  - Mons Pubis
  - Labia Majora
  - Pudendal Cleft
  - Vulval Vestibule
  - Interlabial Sulci
  - Bulb of Vestibule
  - Vaginal Orifice
  - Bartholin's Glands
  - Skene's Glands
  - Labia Minora
  - Clitoris
    - Corpus Cavernosum
    - Crus
    - Glans
  - Urethra
    - Urethral Crest
    - Lacunae of Morgagni
    - Urethral Sphincter

Infectious Disease Organisms

1. BACTERIA

Name of Organism	Gram Stain	Shape/ Arrangment	Oxygen Requirements for Growth	Transmission	Disease(s)	Most Efficacious Medication(s) / Treatment
Aeromonas hydrophila	-	Bacilli	Anaerobe	Fecal-Oral Indirect Physical Contact	Septicemia Endocarditis Myonecrosis Meningeal Infection Gastroenteritis Cellulitis Eczema	Chloramphenicol Florenicol Nitrofuran Derivatives Pyrodinecarboxylic Acids Sulfonamide Tetracycline
Bacillus anthracis	+	Bacilli	Anaerobe	Airborne Direct Physical Contact Fecal-Oral	Cutaneous Anthrax Inhalation Anthrax Gastrointestinal Anthrax	Ciprofloxacin Doxycycline Penicillin
Bacillus cereus	+	Bacilli	Anaerobe	Fecal-Oral Indirect Physical Contact	Food Poisoning Keratitis	Ciprofloxacin Clindamycin Imipenem Meropenem Vancomycin
Bacteroides fragilis	-	Bacilli	Anaerobe	Fecal-Oral Vertical	Peritonitis Septicaemia	Ampicillin-Sulbactam Ertapenem Imipenem-Cilastatin Meropenem Metronidazol Piperacillin-Tazobactam, Tigecycline
Bordetella pertussis	-	Coccobacilli	Aerobe	Droplet Contact Indirect Physical Contact	Pertussis	Azithromycin Clarithromycin
Borrelia burgdorferi	-	Spirochete	Microaerophile	Arthropod Vector	Lyme Disease	Amoxicillin Ceruroxime Doxycycline

Name of Organism	Gram Stain	Shape/ Arrangment	Oxygen Requirements for Growth	Transmission	Disease(s)	Most Efficacious Medication(s) / Treatment
Brucella melitensis	-	Coccobacilli	Aerobe	Airborne Direct Physical Contact	Brucellosis	TMP-SMX
Campylobacter jejuni	-	Helical-Bacilli	Microaerophile	Fecal-Oral	Enteritis Septic Arthritis Meningitis Proctocolitis Guillain-Barre Syndrome	Ciprofloxacin Levofloxacin Moxifloxacin
Citrobacter diversus	-	Bacilli	Anaerobe	Vertical	Neonatal Meningitis Sepsis	Cefepime Ertapenem Gentamicin Imipenem Meropenem Tobramycin
Citrobacter freundii	-	Bacilli	Anaerobe	Direct Physical Contact Fecal-Oral Vertical	Sepsis Gastrointestinal Infection	Cefepime Ertapenem Gentamicin Imipenem Meropenem Tobramycin
Clostridium botulinum	+	Bacilli	Anaerobe	Fecal-Oral Indirect Physical Contact	Botulism	Heptavalent (A,B,C,D,E,F,G) Botulinum Antitoxin Trivalent (A,B,E) Botulinum Antitoxin
Clostridium difficile	+	Bacilli	Anaerobe	Direct Physical Contact Fecal-Oral Indirect Physical Contact	Antibiotic Associated Diarrhea (AAD) Pseudomembranous Colitis (PMC) Antibiotic-Associated Colitis (AAC)	Metronidazole
Clostridium perfringens	+	Bacilli	Anaerobe	Airborne Fecal-Oral Indirect Physical Contact	Food Poisoning Gas Gangrene	Penicillin G +/- Clindamycin

Name of Organism	Gram Stain	Shape/ Arrangment	Oxygen Requirements for Growth	Transmission	Disease(s)	Most Efficacious Medication(s) / Treatment
Clostridium septicum	+	Bacilli	Anaerobe	Airborne Indirect Physical Contact	Gas Gangrene Colorectal Cancer	Carbapenems Cephalosporins Metronidazole Penicillin G
Clostridium tetani	+	Bacilli	Anaerobe	Fecal-Oral Indirect Physical Contact	Tetanus	Azithromycin Metronidazole Penicillin G
Corynebacterium diphtheria	+	Bacilli	Anaerobe	Aerosol Droplets	Diphtheria	Erythromycin Penicillin G
Enterobacteriaceae	-	Bacilli	Anaerobe	Fecal-Oral	Meningitis Pneumonia Urinary Tract Infections Septicemia	Cefepime Ertapenem Imipenem Meropenem Piperacillin-Tazobactam + Gentamicin
Escherichia coli	-	Bacilli	Anaerobe	Airborne Direct Physical Contact Fecal-Oral Indirect Physical Contact	rinary Tract Infections Sepsis Meningitis Traveler's Diarrhea Infant Diarrhea Hemorrhagic Colitis Chronic Diarrhea	Cefazolin Cefotaxime Ceftriaxone Cephalexin Gentamicin, Tobramycin
Fusobacterium nucleatum	-	Spindle-Bacilli	Anaerobe	Direct Physical Contact	Dental Infections Brain Abscesses Chronic Sinusitis Lung Abscesses Aspiration Pneumonia Lemierre's Syndrome	Cephalosporins Clindamycin Metronidazole Penicillins
Haemophilus influenza	-	Bacilli	Aerobe	Aerosol Droplets	Bacterial Meningitis Pneumonia Bronchitis Endocarditis Conjunctivitis Acute Sinusitis Urethritis Ear Infections	Augmentin Azithromycin Cefotaxime, Ceftriaxone Ceftizoxime Clarithromycin Oral 3rd generation Cephalosporins TMP-SMX

Name of Organism	Gram Stain	Shape/ Arrangment	Oxygen Requirements for Growth	Transmission	Disease(s)	Most Efficacious Medication(s) / Treatment
Helicobacter pylori	-	Spindle-Bacilli	Aerobe	Direct Physical Contact Fecal-Oral	Duodenal Ulcers Stomach Cancer Gastritis Peptic Ulcers	Omeprazole + Clarithromycin; Lansoprazole + Amoxicillin + Clarithromycin; Ranitidine Bismuth Citrate + Clarithromycin; Omeprazole + Clarithromycin + Amoxicillin; Bismuth Subsalicylate + Metronidazole + Tetracycline + H2 Receptor Antagonist
Klebsiella pneumoniae	-	Bacilli	Anaerobe	Aerosol Droplets Direct Physical Contact Indirect Physical Contact	Nosocomial Infections Pneumonia Bronchitis Empyema Urinary Tract Infections Thrombophlebitis Septicemia Meningitis	Cefotaxime Ceftizoxime Ceftriaxone Gentamicin Tobramycin
Legionella pneumophila	-	Bacilli	Aerobe	Airborne	Legionnaires' disease Pontiac fever	Azithromycin Ciprofloxacin Clarithromycin Erythromycin Levofloxacin Moxifloxacin
Listeria monocytogenes	-	Bacilli	Anaerobe	Fecal-Oral Indirect Physical Contact	Septicemia Meningitis Encephalitis	Ampicillin TMP-SMX
Mycobacterium leprae	+	Bacilli	Anaerobe	Aerosol Droplets Direct Physical Contact Indirect Physical Contact	Lepromatous Leprosy Tuberculoid Leprosy	Clofazimine Dapsone, Rifampin

Name of Organism	Gram Stain	Shape/ Arrangment	Oxygen Requirements for Growth	Transmission	Disease(s)	Most Efficacious Medication(s) / Treatment
Mycobacterium tuberculosis	+	Bacilli	Aerobe	Airborne Aerosol Droplet Direct Physical Contact	Tuberculosis	Ethambutol Isoniazid Pyrazinamide Rifampin
Neisseria gonorrhoeae	+	Diplococci	Aerobe	Direct Physical Contact Vertical Indirect Physical Contact	Gonorrhea Endometritis Epididymitis Pelvic Inflammatory Disease Proctitis Pharyngitis Conjunctivitis Peritonitis Perihepatitis	Cefixime Ceftriaxone
Neisseria meningitides	-	Diplococci	Aerobe	Direct Physical Contact Droplet Contact	Meningitis Fulminant Sepsis	Cefotaxime Ceftriaxone Pencillin G
Nocardia asteroides	-	Bacilli	Aerobe	Aerosal Droplets Indirect Physical Contact	Pulmonary Nocardiosis Systemic Nocardiosis	Ampicillin Co-Trimoxazole Erythromycin Minocycline Sulfonamides
Proteus mirabilis	+	Bacilli	Anaerobe	Direct Physical Contact Indirect Physical Contact	Urinary Tract Infections Kidney Stones	Amoxicillin Ampicillin Cefotaxime Ceftizoxime Ceftriaxone Gentamicin Tobramycin
Pseudomonas aeruginosa	-	Bacilli	Aerobe	Aerosal Droplet Direct Physical Contact Indirect Physical Contact	Nosocomial Infection Pneumonia Wound Sepsis Bacteremia Urinary Tract Infections Corneal Ulcers Swimmers Ear Folliculitis	Amikacin Cefepime Ceftazidime Ciprofloxacin Gentamycin Imipenem Meropenem Piperacillin-Tazobactam Tobramycin

Name of Organism	Gram Stain	Shape/ Arrangment	Oxygen Requirements for Growth	Transmission	Disease(s)	Most Efficacious Medication(s) / Treatment
Salmonella enteritidis	-	Bacilli	Anaerobe	Airborne Direct Physical Contact Indirect Physical Contact Fecal-Oral	Salmonellosis Food Poisoning Gastroenteritis	Ampicillin Ciprofloxacin
Salmonella typhi	-	Bacilli	Anaerobe	Fecal-Oral	Typhoid Fever	Ceftizoxime Ceftriaxone Ciprofloxacin
Shigella dysenteriae	-	Bacilli	Anaerobe	Direct Physical Contact Fecal-Oral	Dysentery	Ciprofloxacin Levofloxacin
Staphylococcus aureus	-	Cocci	Anaerobe	Direct Physical Contact Indirect Physical Contact Aerosal Droplet	Nosocomial Infection Toxic Shock Syndrome Food Poisoning Scalded Skin Syndrome Abscesses	Cefazolin Cephalexin Dicloxacillin Nafcillin Oxacillin
Staphylococcus aureus (Methicillin-Resitant) MRSA	+	Cocci	Aerobe	Direct Physical Contact Indirect Physical Contact	Abscesses Cellulitits Endocarditis Necrotizing Fasciitis Necrotizing Pneumonia Pyomyositis	Daptomycin Linezolid Vancomycin
Staphylococcus epidermidis	+	Cocci	Anaerobe	Direct Physical Contact Droplet Contact Indirect Physical Contact	Nosocomial Infections Urinary Tract Infections Endocarditis Septicemia	Vancomycin +/- Rifampin
Staphylococcus epidermidis (Methicillin-Resistant) MRSE	+	Cocci	Aerobe	Direct Physical Contact Droplet Contact Indirect Physical Contact	Nosocomial Infections Urinary Tract Infections Endocarditis Septicemia	Vancomycin +/- Gentamicin

Name of Organism	Gram Stain	Shape/ Arrangment	Oxygen Requirements for Growth	Transmission	Disease(s)	Most Efficacious Medication(s) / Treatment
Streptococcus agalactiae (Group B)	+	Streptococci	Anaerobe	Vertical	Neonatal Meningitis Pneumonia Septic Shock Septicemia Meningitis	Amoxicillin Ampicillin Penicillin
Streptococcus mutans	+	Streptococci	Anaerobe	Direct Physical Contact Indirect Physical Contact	Endocardititis Tooth Decay	Bacitracin Polymyxin B
Streptococcus pneumoniae	+	Streptococci	Anaerobe	Direct Physical Contact Droplet Contact	Acute Sinusitis Brain Abscess Cellulitis Otitis Media Meningitis Bacteremia Sepsis Osteomyelitis Septic Arthritis Endocarditis Peritonitis Pericarditis	Amoxicillin Ampicillin Penicillin G or V
Streptococcus pneumonia (Penicillin-Resistant)	+	Streptococci	Aerobe	Direct Physical Contact Droplet Contact	Acute Sinusitis Brain Abscess Cellulitis Otitis Media Meningitis Bacteremia Sepsis Osteomyelitis Septic Arthritis Endocarditis Peritonitis Pericarditis	Levofloxacin Moxifloxacin Telithromycin Vancomycin
Streptococcus pyogenes (Group A)	+	Streptococci	Anaerobe	Direct Physical Contact Droplet Contact	Strep Throat Impetigo Necrotizing Fasciitis Streptococcal Toxic Shock Syndrome	Amoxicillin Ampicillin Penicillin G or V

Name of Organism	Gram Stain	Shape/ Arrangment	Oxygen Requirements for Growth	Transmission	Disease(s)	Most Efficacious Medication(s) / Treatment
Treponema pallidum	-	Spirochete	Microaerophile	Direct Physical Contact	Syphilis Bejel Pinta Yaws	Penicillin G
Vibrio cholerae	-	Bacilli	Aerobe	Fecal-Oral	Cholera	Doxycycline
Yesinia pestis	-	Coccobacilli	Anaerobe	Arthropod Vector Direct Physical Contact Droplet Contact	Pneumonic Plague Septicemic Plague Bubonic Plague	Chloramphenicol Doxycycline Fluoroquinolones Gentamicin Streptomycin Tetracycline

2. PARASITES

Name of Organism	Transmission	Disease(s)	Most Efficacious Medication(s) / Treatment
Acanthamoeba (Amoeba)	Indirect physical contact, Fecal-oral	*Acanthamoeba* keratitis, Granulomatous Amebic Encephalitis (GAE), Disseminated infection	Rifampicin, Trimethroprim-sulfamethoxazole, Ketokonazole, Fluconazole, Sulfadiazine, Miconazole, Itraconazole, Pentamidine, Flucytosine, Propamidine isethionate, Chlorhexidine, Natamycin
Ancylostoma duodenale (Old World hookworm)	Indirect physical contact, Fecal-oral	Ancylostomiasis, Geophagy, Protein deficiency, Iron deficiency anemia	Albendazole, Mebendazole, Pyrantel
Anisakis (Roundworm)	Fecal-oral	Gastric anisakiasis, Enteric anisakiasis, Intestinal anisakiasis, Intestinal obstruction, Appendicitis, Peritonitis, Allergic reaction	Albendazole
Archiacanthocephala (Parasitic worm)	Fecal-oral	Anemia	Ivermectin, Loperamid

Name of Organism	Transmission	Disease(s)	Most Efficacious Medication(s) / Treatment
Ascaris lumbricoides (Roundworm)	Indirect physical contact, Fecal-oral	Ascariasis, Parasitic pneumonia, Löffler's syndrome	Mebendazole, Nitazoxanide, Ivermectin, Albendazole, Pyrantel pamoate
Babesia microti (*Ixodes* ticks)	Arthropod vector	Babesiosis, Hemolytic anemia	Atovaquone, Azithromycin, Clindamycin, Quinine
Balantidium coli (Ciliate protozoan)	Fecal-oral	Balantidiasis	Tetracyclines, Metronidazole, Iodoquinol
Baylisascaris procyonis (Roundworm)	Fecal-oral	Baylisascariasis	Albendazole
Blastocystis hominis (Protozoan)	Fecal-oral, Indirect physical contact	Blastocystosis	Metronidazole, Trimethoprim (TMP), Sulfamethoxazole (SMX), Nitazoxanide, Flagyl, Bactrim, Septra, Yodoxin
Brugia malayi (Mosquito, Roundworm)	Arthropod vector	Lymphatic filariasis	Diethylcarbamazine, Albendazole-DEC, Albendazole-ivermectin, Tetracyclines, Rifampicin, Chloramphenicol
Brugia timori (Mosquito, Roundworm)	Arthropod vector	Timor filariasis	Diethylcarbamazine, Albendazole
Calliphoridae (Bow fly)	Arthropod vector	Myiasis, Dysentery, Flystrike, Salmonellosis	Petroleum jelly
Cestoda (Tapeworm)	Fecal-oral	Cysticercosis	Albendazole, Praziquantel
Cimex lectularius (Bed bug)	Arthropod vector	Allergic reaction, Anemia	Topical hydrocortisone, Benadryl
Clonorchis sinensis (Chinese liver fluke)	Fecal-oral	Clonorchiasis	Triclabendazole, Praziquantel, Bithionol, Albendazole, Mebendazole
Cochliomyia hominivorax (Screwworm)	Arthropod vector, Indirect physical contact	Skin wounds	Ivermectin, Nitrofurazone
Cryptosporidium (*Coccidia*)	Fecal-oral, Direct physical contact, Indirect physical contact	Cryptosporidiosis	Nitazoxanide
Demodex folliculorum (Mite)	Direct physical contact	Demodicosis, Roseaceous skin rash, Acne, Blackheads	Erythromycin ophthalmic, Mercury oxide 1% ointment, Pilocarpine 4% gel

Name of Organism	Transmission	Disease(s)	Most Efficacious Medication(s) / Treatment
Dermatobia hominis (Human botfly)	Arthropod vector	Wound myiasis, Furuncular myiasis, Nasopharyngeal myiasis, Ophthalmomyiasis, Intestinal myiasis, Urogenital myiasis, Hematophagous myiasis	Ivermectin
Dicrocoelium dendriticum (Lancet liver fluke)	Fecal-oral	Biliary colic, Bloating, Diarrhea, Hepatomegaly, Cirrhosis, Urticaria	Praziquantel, Triclobendazole, Mirazid
Dientamoeba fragilis (Amoeba)	Fecal-oral	Dientamoebiasis, Travellers diarrhea, Chronic diarrhea, Fatigue, Failure to thrive	Metronidazole, Iodoquinol, Paromomycin
Dioctophyme renale (Giant kidney worm)	Fecal-oral	*Dioctophyme* renalis infection, Hematuria, Nephritis, Loin pain, Renal enlargement, Renal colic	Surgical excision
Diphyllobothrium latum (Broad fish tapeworm)	Fecal-oral	Diphyllobothriasis, Diarrhea, Abdominal pain, Vomiting, Weight loss, Fatigue, Constipation, B_{12} deficiency, Megaloblastic anemia	Praziquantel, Niclosamide
Dracunculus medinensis (Guinea worm)	Fecal-oral	Dracunculiasis, Nausea, Vomiting, Fever, Cellulitis, Abscesses, Sepsis, Septic Arthritis, Contractures, Tetanus	Manual removal of worm
Echinococcus granulosus (Hyper tapeworm)	Fecal-oral	Cystic echinococcosis	Albendazole, Chemotherapy, Cyst puncture, Percutaneous aspiration injection of chemicals and reaspiration (PAIR)

Name of Organism	Transmission	Disease(s)	Most Efficacious Medication(s) / Treatment
Echinococcus multilocularis (Tapeworm)	Fecal-oral	Alveolar echinococcosis	Surgery with long term chemotherapy, Mebendazole, Albendazole
Echinostoma echinatum (Trematode fluke)	Fecal-oral	Human echinostomiasis	Praziquantel, Mebendazole, Albendazole, Niclosamide, Tetrachloroethylene
Entamoeba histolytica (Amoeba)	Fecal-oral, Direct physical contact	Intestinal amoebiasis, Extra-intestinal amoebiasis Amoebic dysentery	Iodoquinol, Paromomycin, Diloxanide furoate, Metronidazole
Enterobius vermicularis (Pinworm)	Fecal-oral, Direct physical contact, Indirect physical contact	Enterobiasis	Mebendazole, Pyrantel pamoate, Albendazole
Fasciola gigantica (Giant liver fluke)	Fecal-oral	Fascioliasis	Triclabendazole
Fasciola hepatica (Common liver fluke)	Fecal-oral	Fasciolosis	Triclabendazole
Fasciolopsis buski (Giant intestinal fluke)	Fecal-oral	Fasciolopsiasis	Praziquantel
Giardia lamblia (Protozoan)	Fecal-oral, Indirect physical contact, Direct physical contactl	Giardiasis	Metronidazole, Tinidazole, Nitazoxanide
Gnathostoma hispidum (Roundworm)	Fecal-oral	Gnathostomiasis	Albendazole, Ivermectin
Gnathostoma spinigerum (Roundworm)	Fecal-oral	Gnathostomiasis	Albendazole, Ivermectin
Hymenolepis diminuta (Rat tapeworm)	Fecal-oral, Indirect physical contact	Hymenolepiasis	Praziquantel
Hymenolepis nana (Dwarf tapeworm)	Fecal-oral, Indirect physical contact	Hymenolepiasis	Praziquantel
Isospora belli (Coccidia)	Fecal-oral, Indirect physical contact, Direct physical contact	Cystoisosporiasis	Trimethoprim-sulfamethoxazole
Leishmania (Sandflies)	Arthropod vector	Cutaneous leishmaniasis, Visceral leishmaniasis, Mucocutaneous leishmaniasis	Sodium stibogluconate, Meglumine antimoniate, Liposomal amphotericin B, Fluconazole, Ketoconazole, Itraconazole
Linguatula serrate (Tongue worm)	Fecal-oral	Halzoun Syndrome, Linguatulosis	Surgical removal, Praziquantel

Name of Organism	Transmission	Disease(s)	Most Efficacious Medication(s) / Treatment
Loa loa filarial (Eye worm, Deer fly)	Arthropod vector	*Loa loa* filariasis	Diethylcarbamazine (DEC), Ivermectin
Mansonella streptocerca (Midge)	Arthropod vector	Streptocerciasis	Ivermectin
Metagonimus yokogawai (Japanese intestinal fluke)	Fecal-oral	Metagonimiasis	Praziquantel
Naegleria fowleri (Brain eating amoeba)	Nasal insufflation	Primary amoebic meningoencephalitis (PAM)	Amphotericin B, Fluconazole, Rifampicin
Necator americanus (New World hookworm)	Indirect physical contact	Necatoriasis	Albendazole, Mebendazole, Tetrachloroethene
Oestroidea (Bot fly)	Arthropod vector	Cutaneous Myiasis, Nasal Myiasis, Aural Myiasis, Ophthalmomyiasis	Petroleum jelly
Onchocerca volvulus (Black fly, Filarial nematode)	Arthropod vector	Onchocerciasis, Subcutaneous filariasis	Ivermectin, Doxycycline
Opisthorchis viverrini (Southeaset Asian liver fluke)	Fecal-oral	Opisthorchiasis, Cholangiocarcinoma	Praziquantel, Albendazole
Paragonimus westermani (Lung fluke)	Fecal-oral	Paragonimiasis	Praziquantel, Triclabendazole, Bithionol
Pediculus humanus (Head lice)	Arthropod vector, Direct physical contact, Indirect physical contact	Pediculosis, Pruritus	Pyrethrin with Piperonyl butoxide, Malathion lotion, Benzyl alcohol lotion
Pediculus humanus corporis (Body lice)	Arthropod vector, Direct physical contact, Indirect physical contact	Pediculosis, Pruritus, Vagabond's disease, Epidemic typhus, Trench fever, Epidemic relapsing fever	Pyrethrin with Piperonyl butoxide, Malathion lotion, Benzyl alcohol lotion
Phthirus pubis (Pubic lice)	Arthropod vector, Direct physical contact, Indirect physical contact	Pediculosis	Pyrethrin with Piperonyl butoxide, Permethrin lotion
Plasmodium falciparum (*Anopheles* mosquito)	Arthropod vector, Vertical, Blood transfusion	Malaria (*P.f.* malignant tertian malaria)	Chloroquine, Atovaquone-proguanil, Artemether-lumefantrine, Mefloquine, Quinine, Quinidine, Doxycycline, Clindamycin

Name of Organism	Transmission	Disease(s)	Most Efficacious Medication(s) / Treatment
Plasmodium knowlesi (*Anopheles* mosquito)	Arthropod vector, Vertical, Blood transfusion, Monkey bite	Malaria (*P.k.* severe quotidian malaria)	Chloroquine, Hydroxychloroquine
Plasmodium malariae (*Anopheles* mosquito)	Arthropod vector, Vertical, Blood transfusion	Malaria (*P.m.* benign quartan malaria)	Chloroquine, Hydroxychloroquine
Plasmodium ovale (*Anopheles* mosquito)	Arthropod vector, Vertical, Blood transfusion	Malaria (*P.o.* benign tertian malaria)	Chloroquine, Hydroxychloroquine
Plasmodium vivax (*Anopheles* mosquito)	Arthropod vector, Vertical, Blood transfusion	Malaria (*P.v.* benign tertian malaria)	Chloroquine, Hydroxychloroquine, Quinine sulfate with Doxycycline, Tetracycline, Atovaquone-proguanil, Mefloquine
Rhinosporidium seeberi (Eukaryote)	Nasal insufflation, Indirect physical contact	Rhinosporidiosis	Surgical excision, Dapsone
Sarcophagidae (Flesh fly)	Arthropod vector	Myiasis, Leprosy, Intestinal pseudomyiasis, Blood poisoning	Petroleum jelly
Sarcoptes scabiei (Human itch mite)	Arthropod vector, Direct physical contact, Indirect physical contact	Scabies, Post-streptococcal glomerulonephritis	Permethrin cream 5%, Crotamiton cream 10%, Lindane lotion 1%, Ivermectin
Schistosoma haematobium (Human blood fluke)	Direct contact	Urinary schistosomiasis	Praziquantel
Schistosoma japonicum (Human blood fluke)	Direct contact	Intestinal schistosomiasis	Praziquantel
Schistosoma mansoni (Human blood fluke)	Direct contact	Intestinal schistosomiasis	Praziquantel
Schistosoma mekongi (Human blood fluke)	Direct contact	Asian Intestinal schistosomiasis	Praziquantel
Spirometra erinaceieuropaei (Tapeworm)	Fecal-oral, Indirect physical contact	Sparganosis	Surgical removal, Praziquantel

Name of Organism	Transmission	Disease(s)	Most Efficacious Medication(s) / Treatment
Strongyloides stercoralis (Threadworm)	Direct physical contact, Indirect physical contact	Strongyloidiasis, Hyperinfection syndrome, Disseminated strongyloidiasis	Ivermectin, Albendazole
Taenia saginata (Beef tapeworm)	Fecal-oral	Cysticercosis	Praziquantel, Niclosamide
Taenia solium (Pork tapeworm)	Fecal-oral	Cysticercosis	Praziquantel, Niclosamide
Toxocara canis (Dog roundworm)	Fecal-oral, Indirect physical contact	Ocular toxocariasis, Visceral toxocariasis	Albendazole, Mebendazole
Toxoplasma gondii (Protozoan)	Fecal-oral, Indirect physical contact, Direct physical contact, Vertical	Toxoplasmosis, Retinochoroiditis	Pyrimethamine, Sulfadiazine, Leucovorin, Clindamycin, Trimethoprim, Sulfamethoxazole
Trichinella britovi (Roundworm)	Fecal-oral	Trichinosis	Albendazole, Mebendazole
Trichinella spiralis (Pork roundworm)	Fecal-oral	Trichinosis	Albendazole, Mebendazole
Trichobilharzia regent (Avian blood fluke)	Direct physical contact, Indirect physical contact	Swimmer's itch	Hydroxyzine
Trichomonas vaginalis (Protozoan)	Direct physical contact	Trichomoniasis	Metronidazole, Tinidazole
Trichuris trichiura (Whipworm)	Fecal-oral, Indirect physical contact	Trichuriasis	Albendazole, Mebendazole, Ivermectin
Trypanosoma brucei (Tsetse fly)	Arthopod vector	Sleeping sickness	Suramin, Melarsoprol, Pentamidine, Eflornithine
Trypanosoma cruzi (Triatomine bug)	Arthropod vector, Vertical, Direct physical contact, Indirect physical contact	Chagas disease	Benznidazole, Nifurtimox
Tunga penetrans (Chigoe flea)	Arthropod vector	Tungiasis	Ivermectin, Metrifonate
Wuchereria bancrofti (*Anopheles* mosquito, roundworm)	Arthropod vector	Elephantiasis, Lymphatic filariasis, lymphatic system	Diethylcarbamazine (DEC), Ivermectin, Albendazole

3. VIRUSES

Name of Organism	Transmission	Disease(s)	Most Efficacious Medication(s) / Treatment
Adenovirus (Non-enveloped)	Droplet contact, Fecal-oral, Direct physical contact	Acute febrile pharyngitis, Pharyngoconjunctival fever, Epidemic keratoconjunctivitis, Infantile gastroenteritis	(Drugs for symptomatic treatment) Cidofovir, Ribavirin, Ganciclovir, Vidarabine
Coxsackie virus (Non-enveloped)	Fecal-oral, Droplet contact	Coxsackie infections, Hand foot and& mouth disease, Conjunctivitis, Pleurodynia, Meningitis, Myocarditis, Pericarditis	(Drugs for symptomatic treatment) Acetaminophen, Diphenhydramine, Benadryl
Epstein-Barr virus (Enveloped)	Direct physical contact	Infectious mononucleosis, Burkitt's lymphoma	(Drugs for symptomatic treatment) Nonsteroidal anti-inflammatory drugs, Corticosteroid injections
Hepatitis A virus (Non-enveloped)	Fecal-oral, Direct physical contact	Acute hepatitis	None
Hepatitis B virus (Enveloped)	Direct physical contact, Indirect physical contact	Acute hepatitis, Chronic hepatitis, Hepatic cirrhosis, Hepatocellular carcinoma	Adefovir, Entecavir, Lamivudine, Pegylated (PEG) interferon Alpha-2a, Telbivudine, Tenofovir
Hepatitis C virus (Enveloped)	Direct physical contact, Indirect physical contact, Vertical	Acute hepatitis, Chronic hepatitis, Hepatic cirrhosis, Hepatocellular carcinoma	Pegylated (PEG) interferon Alpha-2b+, Ribavarin

Name of Organism	Transmission	Disease(s)	Most Efficacious Medication(s) / Treatment
Herpes simplex virus, type 1 (Enveloped)	Direct physical contact, Vertical	Gingivostomatitis, tonsillitis, pharyngitis, keratoconjunctivitis, Herpes labialis, Cold sores, Eczema herpetiform	Acyclovir, Famciclovir, Foscarnet, Penciclovir, Valaciclovir
Herpes simplex virus, type 2 (Enveloped)	Direct physical contact, Vertical	Genital herpes, Neonatal herpes, Genital ulcer disease, Aseptic meningitis, Eczema herpetiform	Acyclovir, Famciclovir, Foscarnet, Penciclovir, Cidofovir, Valaciclovir, Docosanol
Cytomegalovirus (Enveloped)	Direct physical contact, Vertical	Infectious mononucleosis, Cytomegalic inclusion disease, Congenital cytomegalovirus infection	Ganciclovir, Cidofovir, Foscarnet, Valganciclovir, Leflunomide, Cytomegalovirus immune globulin
Human herpes virus, type 8 (Enveloped)	Direct physical contact, Vertical	Kaposi sarcoma, Multicentric Castleman disease, Primary effusion lymphoma	Ganciclovir
HIV (Enveloped)	Direct physical contact, Vertical	AIDS	HAART
Influenza virus (Enveloped)	Droplet contact	Influenza (H_1N_1, H_1N_2, H_3N_2), Reye syndrome	Rimantadine, Zanamivir, Oseltamivir, Amantadine
Measles virus (Enveloped)	Droplet contact, Direct physical contact, Indirect physical contact	Measles, Post-infectious encephalomyelitis	(Drugs for symptomatic treatment) Acetaminophen, Ibuprofen, Naproxen, Vitamin A, Preventative—Measles vaccine
Mumps virus (Enveloped)	Droplet contact, Direct physical contact	Mumps, Sensorineural hearing loss, Encephalitis	(Drugs for symptomatic treatment) Acetaminophen, Ibuprofen, Preventative—Mumps vaccine

Name of Organism	Transmission	Disease(s)	Most Efficacious Medication(s) / Treatment
Human papillomavirus (Non-enveloped)	Direct contact	Hyperplastic epithelial lesions, Cervical carcinoma, Squamous cell carcinomas	Liquid nitrogen, Laser vaporization, Cytotoxic chemicals, Interferon, Cidofovir
Parainfluenza virus (Enveloped)	Droplet contact	Croup, Pneumonia, Bronchiolitis, Pneumonia, Common cold, Respiratory tract infection	Ribavirin, Dexamethasone, Budesonide inhaled, Prednisone, Prednisolone, Epinephrine racemic
Poliovirus (Non-enveloped)	Fecal-oral	Poliomyelitis	(Drugs for symptomatic treatment) Acetaminophen, Nonsteroidal anti-inflammatory agents, Preventative—Polio vaccine
Rabies virus (Enveloped)	Animal bite, Droplet contact	Rabies	Rabies vaccine, Rabies immunoglobulin
Respiratory syncytial virus (Enveloped)	Droplet contact, Fecal-oral, Direct physical contact, Indirect physical contact	Bronchiolitis, Pneumonia, Acute respiratory infection	Ribavirin, Palivizumab, Albuterol, Alupent, Combivent, Maxair, Xopenex
Rubella virus (Enveloped)	Droplet contact	German measles, Congenital rubella syndrome	(Drugs for symptomatic treatment) Acetominophen, Preventative—Rubella vaccine
Varicella-zoster virus (Enveloped)	Droplet contact	Varicella, Herpes zoster	Acyclovir, Famciclovir, Valacyclovir, VZV immune globulin, Zoster-immune globulin (ZIG), Vidarabine

4. FUNGI

Name of Organism	Transmission	Disease(s)	Most Efficacious Medication(s) / Treatment
Absidia corymbifera	Aerosol	Zygomycosis, Mucormycosis, Phycomycosis, Basidiobolomycosis	Amphotericin B
Aspergillus fumigatus	Aerosol, Indirect physical contact	Invasive aspergillosis, Allergic aspergillosis, Chronic pulmonary aspergillosis	Amphotericin B, Voriconazole, Caspofungin, Prednisone, Itraconazole
Basidiobolus ranarum	Aerosol, Arthropod vector	Basidiobolomycosis, Subcutaneous zygomycosis, Mycotic dermatitis	Itraconazole
Blastomyces dermatitidis	Aerosol	Cutaneous blastomycosis, Osseous blastomycosis	Posaconazole, Amphotericin B, Itraconazole
Candida albicans	Direct physical contact, Vertical	Oral thrush, Vaginitis, Candidemia, Esophageal candidiasis	Voriconazole, Amphotericin B, Caspofungin, Fluconazole, Topical azole
Coccidioides immitis	Aerosol	Primary pulmonary coccidioidomycosis, Disseminated coccidioidomycosis, Primary cutaneous coccidioidomycosis	Voriconazole, Ketoconazole, Itraconazole, Fluconazole, Amphotericin B
Coccidioides posadasii	Aerosol	Primary pulmonary coccidioidomycosis, Disseminated coccidioidomycosis, Primary cutaneous coccidioidomycosis	Voriconazole, Amphotericin B, Fluconazole, Itraconazole, Ketoconazole
Cryptococcus neoformans	Aerosol	Cutaneous cryptococcosis Pulmonary cryptococcosis, Cryptococcal meningitis	Amphotericin B, Flucytosine

Name of Organism	Transmission	Disease(s)	Most Efficacious Medication(s) / Treatment
Epidermophyton floccosum	Direct physical contact, Indirect physical contact	Tinea pedis, Tinea cruris, Tinea capitis, Tinea corporis, Onychomycosis	Fluconazole, Ketoconazole, Itraconazole, Voriconazole, Naftifine, Terbinafine, Butenafine, Chlotriminazole
Exophiala werneckii	Indirect physical contact	Tinea nigra	Amphotericin B, Ketoconazole, Miconazole, Clotrimazole, Tretinoin, Salicylic acid, Ciclopirox
Fonsecaea compacta	Indirect physical contact	Chromoblastomycosis	Voriconazole, Itraconazole, Terbinafine, Flucytosine
Fusarium oxysporum	Indirect physical contact	Fusarium keratitis, Onychomycosis, Hyalohyphomycosis	Voriconazole, Natamycin, Fluconazole, Amphotericin B, Terbinafine, Itraconazole, Ciclopirox, Amorolfine
Histoplasma capsulatum	Aerosol	Primary pulmonary histoplasmosis, Progressive disseminated histoplasmosis, Primary cutaneous histoplasmosis, African histoplasmosis	Posaconazole, Amphotericin B, Itraconazole
Lacazia loboi	Indirect physical contact	Lobomycosis	Cryosurgery, Clofazimine, Dapsone
Malassezia furfur	Indirect physical contact	Seborrheic dermatitis, Folliculitis, Pityriasis versicolor, Atopic dermatitis	Itraconazole, Ciclopirox, Ketoconazole, Econazole, Selenium sulfide topical
Microsporum canis	Direct physical contact, Indirect physical contact	Tinea capitis	Griseofulvin, Fluconazole, Terbinafine, Itraconazole
Paracoccidioides brasiliensis	Indirect physical contact, Aerosol	Paracoccidioidomycosis	Sulfadimethoxime, Sulfadiazine, Co-trimoxazole, Amphotericin B, Ketoconazole

Name of Organism	Transmission	Disease(s)	Most Efficacious Medication(s) / Treatment
Penicillium marneffei	Aerosol	Penicilliosis	Amphotericin B, Itraconazole, Voriconazole, Ketoconazole, Miconazole, Flucytosine
Phialophora parasitica	Indirect physical contact	Chromoblastomycosis, Phaeohyphomycosis	Amphotericin B, Fluconazole, Itraconazole, Terbinafine, Voriconazole
Piedraia hortae	Direct physical contact, Indirect physical contact	Black piedra, Trichosporosis	Terbinafine
Pneumocystis jirovecii	Aerosol, Indirect physical contact	Pneumocystis pneumonia	Co-trimoxazole, Pentamidine, Trimetrexate, Dapsone, Atovaquone, Primaquine, Clindamycin
Rhizopus arrhizus	Aerosol, Indirect physical contact, Oral	Mucormycosis	Caspofungin, Amphotericin B, Posaconazole
Sporothrix schenckii	Indirect physical contact, Animal bite	Cutaneous sporotrichosis, Pulmonary sporotrichosis, Disseminated sporotrichosis	Voriconazole, Potassium iodide, Itraconazole, Fluconazole, Amphotericin B
Trichophyton rubrum	Indirect physical contact, Direct physical contact	Athlete's foot, Jock itch, Ringworm	Miconazole, Terbinafine, Clotrimazole, Ketoconazole, Tolnaftate, Nystatin, Fluconazole
Trichosporon beigelii	Direct physical contact, Indirect physical contact	White piedra, Trichosporonosis	Posaconazole, Voriconazole, Amphotericin B, Fluconazole, Flucytosine, Caspofungin, Micafungin

Common Medical Abbreviations

1. ACRONYMS FOR COMMON DISEASES AND DISORDERS

Acronym	Common Diseases and Disorders
AAA	Abdominal Aortic Aneurysm
ACD	Autosomal Chromosome Disorders
ACS	Acute Coronary Syndrome
AD	Alzheimer's Disease
ADD	Attention Deficit Disorder
ADHD	Attention Deficit Hyperactivity Disorder
AF	Atrial Fibrillation
AIDS	Acquired Immune Deficiency Syndrome
ALL	Acute Lymphoblastic Leukemia
ALS	Amyotrophic Lateral Sclerosis
ARDS	Acute Respiratory Distress Syndrome
ARF	Acute Renal Failure
AS	Asperger Syndrome
ASDs	Autism Spectrum Disorders
BD	Bipolar Disorder
BDD	Body Dysmorphic Disorder
BEH	Behaviorally/Emotionally Handicapped
BPD	Borderline Personality Disorder
BPH	Benign Prostatic Hyperplasia
BV	Bacterial Vaginosis
CA	Cancer
CAD	Coronary Artery Disease
CAPD	Central Auditory Processing Disorder

Acronym	Common Diseases and Disorders
CF	Cystic Fibrosis
CFS	Chronic Fatigue Syndrome
CHD	Congenital Heart Disease
CHD	Coronary Heart Disease
CHF	Congestive Heart Failure
CKD	Chronic Kidney Disease
COPD	Chronic Obstructive Pulmonary Disease
CP	Cerebral Palsy
CRF	Chronic Renal Failure
CRPS	Complex Regional Pain Syndrome
CTS	Carpal Tunnel Syndrome
CVD	Cardiovascular Disease
DD	Developmental Disability
DH	Developmentally Handicapped
DI	Diabetes Insipidus
DID	Dissociative Identity Disorder
DJD	Degenerative Joint Disease
DKA	Diabetic Ketoacidosis
DM	Diabetes Mellitus
DMD	Duchenne Muscular Dystrophy
DRSP	Drug-Resistant Streptococcus Pneumoniae
DU	Duodenal Ulcer
DUB	Dysfunctional Uterine Bleeding
DS	Down Syndrome
DVT	Deep Vein Thrombosis
ED	Emotionally Disturbed
ED	Erectile Dysfunction
EDS	Ehlers-Danlos Syndrome
EFAD	Essential Fatty Acid Deficiency
EHK	Epidermolytic Hyperkeratosis

Acronym	Common Diseases and Disorders
FAS	Fetal Alcohol Syndrome
Flu	Influenza
FMA	Focal Muscular Atrophies
FMS	Fibromyalgia Syndrome
GAD	Generalized Anxiety Disorder
GAN	Giant Axonal Neuropathy
GBS	Guillain-Barré Syndrome
GC	Gonorrhea
GD	Gestational Diabetes
GERD	Gastroesophageal Reflux Disease
GIB	Gastrointestinal Bleeding
GN	Glomerulonephritis (Nephritis)
GU	Gastric Ulcer
HAV	Hepatitis A Virus
HBP	High Blood Pressure
HBV	Hepatitis B Virus
HCC	Hepatocellular Carcinoma
HCV	Hepatitis C Virus
HD	Huntington's Disease
HFA	High Functioning Autism
HFMD	Hand, Foot, and Mouth Disease
HI	Hearing Impaired
HIV	Human Immunodeficiency Virus
HPV	Human Papillomavirus Infection
HSV	Herpes Simplex Virus
HTN	Hypertension
IBC	Inflammatory Breast Cancer
IBD	Inflammatory Bowel Disease
IBS	Irritable Bowel Syndrome
IC/PBS	Interstitial Cystitis/Painful Bladder Syndrome

Acronym	Common Diseases and Disorders
ID	Infectious Disease
IDA	Iron Deficiency Anemia
IDDM	Insulin Dependent Diabetes Mellitus
IMN	Infectious Mononucleosis
IMS	Irritable Male Syndrome
INAD	Infantile Neuroaxonal Dystrophy
JHD	Juvenile Huntington's Disease
JIA	Juvenile Idiopathic Arthritis
JRA	Juvenile Rheumatoid Arthritis
LD	Legionnaires' Disease
LDs	Learning Disabilities/Differences
LFA	Low Functioning Autism
LGV	Lymphogranuloma Venereum
MAC	Mycobacterium Avium Complex
MD	Muscular Dystrophy
MDD	Major Depressive Disorder (Clinical Depression)
MMRV	Measles, Mumps, Rubella, Varicella
MND	Motor Neuron Disease
Mono	Infectious Mononucleosis (Glandular Fever)
MR/DD	Mentally Retarded/Developmentally Disabled
MRSA	Methicillin-Resistant Staphylococcus Aureus
MS	Multiple Sclerosis
MSDD	Multi-Sensory Developmental Delays
NAS	Neonatal Abstinence Syndrome
NIDDM	Non-Insulin Dependent Diabetes Mellitus
NLD	Nonverbal Learning Disability
NMS	Neuronal Migration Disorder
NP	Niemann-Pick Disease
NTD	Neural Tube Defect
OA	Osteoarthritis

Acronym	Common Diseases and Disorders
OCD	Obsessive Compulsive Disorder
OCPD	Obsessive Compulsive Personality Disorder
ODD	Oppositional Defiant Disorder
OMA	Ocular Motor Apraxia
OP	Osteoporosis
OSA	Obstructive Sleep Apnea
Osteo	Osteomyelitis
PAD	Peripheral Artery Disease
PBC	Primary Biliary Cirrhosis
PCa	Prostate Cancer
PCOS	Polycystic Ovarian Syndrome
PD	Parkinson's Disease
PDA	Patent Ductus Arteriosis
PDD	Pervasive Developmental Disorder
PKD	Polycystic Kidney Disease
PLS	Primary Lateral Sclerosis
PML	Progressive Multifocal Leukoencephalopathy
PMS	Premenstrual Syndrome
PTSD	Post-Traumatic Stress Disorder
PUD	Peptic Ulcer Disease
RA	Rheumatoid Arthritis
RAD	Reactive Airway Disease
RD	Retinal Detachment
RF	Rheumatic Fever
RLS	Restless Legs Syndrome
RMD	Repetitive Motion Disorder
RS	Reye's Syndrome
RSD	Reflex Sympathetic Dystrophy
RTI	Respiratory Tract Infection
SARS	Severe Acute Respiratory Syndrome

Acronym	Common Diseases and Disorders
SB	Spina Bifida
SBS	Shaken Baby Syndrome
SIDS	Sudden Infant Death Syndrome
SLE	Systemic Lupus Erythematosus
SMA	Spinal Muscular Atrophy
SOB	Shortness of Breath (Dyspnea)
SOD	Septo-Optic Dysplasia
SS	Sickle-Cell Disease (Anemia)
STD	Sexually Transmitted Disease
STI	Sexually Transmitted Infection
Strep	Streptococcus
SVT	Supraventricular Tachycardia
SWS	Sturge-Weber Syndrome
TB	Tuberculosis
TBI	Traumatic Brain Injury
TN	Trigeminal Neuralgia
TOS	Thoracic Outlet Syndrome
TS	Tourette Syndrome
TSC	Tuberous Sclerosis
UC	Ulcerative Colitis
UTI	Urinary Tract Infection
VD	Venereal Disease
VHL	Von Hippel-Lindau Disease
VSD	Ventricular Septal Defect
VV	Varicose Veins
WD	Wilson's Disease
WS	Williams Syndrome
XLSA	X-Linked Sideroblastic Anemia
XP	Xeroderma Pigmentosa
YF	Yellow Fever

2. ABBREVIATIONS FOR COMMON DIAGNOSTIC AND LABORATORY TESTS

Abbreviation	Common Diagnostic and Laboratory Tests
ACP	Anterior Chamber Paracentesis
AFTS	Autonomic Reflex Tests
AMCE	Amniocentesis
AUDMY	Audiometry
AUSC	Auscultation
BAG	Bronchial Arteriography
BLCU	Blood Culture
BLTES	Blood Tests
BMAT	Bone Marrow Aspiration and Trephine Biopsy
BPMS	Blood Pressure Measurements
BRO	Bronchoscopy
Bx	Biopsy
CART	Coronary Arteriography
CBC	Complete Blood Count
CC	Cardiac Catheterization
CC	Cell Culture
CCA	Conventional Chromosome Analysis
COBI	Cone Biopsy
COL	Colonoscopy
COLPY	Colposcopy
CT	Computed Tomography
CVS	Chorionic Villus Sampling
D&C	Dilation and Curettage
DEC	Doppler Echocardiography
DEXA	Dual X-Ray Absorptiometry
DIV	Direct Injection Venography
DLS	Diagnostic Laparoscopy
EAR	Electroencephalographic Audiometry
ECG or EKG	Electrocardiogram

Abbreviation	Common Diagnostic and Laboratory Tests
ECHG	Echocardiography
EEG	Electroencephalogram
ELISA	Enzyme-Linked Immunosorbent Assay
EMB	Endometrial Biopsy
EMG	Electromyography
EN	Endoscopy
ERCP	Endoscopic Retrograde Cholangiopancreatography
ESWL	Extracorporeal Shock Wave Lithotripsy
FNB	Fine-Needle Biopsy
FLSCY	Fluoroscopy
GE	Gastrointestinal Endoscopy
GI	Glycemic Index
GTT	Glucose Tolerance Test
HRU	High-Resolution Ultrasonography
HYS	Hysteroscopy
I&O	Intake and Output
IOA	Intraoperative Arteriography
IVP	Intravenous Urography
JT.ASP.	Joint Aspiration
LAP	Laparoscopy
LASIK	Laser-Assisted In-Situ Keratomileusis
LFT	Liver Function Test
LNB	Large Needle Biopsy
LP	Lumbar Puncture (Spinal Tap)
MESTCY	Mediastinoscopy
MMG	Mammography
MMRI	Micromagnetic Resonance Imaging
MLG	Myelography
MRI	Magnetic Resonance Imaging
MRU	Magnetic Resonance Urography

Abbreviation	Common Diagnostic and Laboratory Tests
NCS	Nerve Conduction Study
OBT	Occult Blood Test
OPSCY	Ophthalmoscopy
P&A	Percussion and Auscultation
PACEN	Paracentesis
Pap	Papanicolaou Test (Pap Smear)
PAT	Preadmission Testing
PET	Positron Emission Tomography
PFT	Pulmonary Function Test
PMG	Pneumomyelography
PTC	Percutaneous Transhepatic Cholangiography
RBCV	Red Blood Cell Venography
SCLT	Sex Chromosome Loss Test
Scope	Microscope or Endoscope
SIG	Sigmoidoscopy
SPMET	Spirometry
SPTAP	Spinal Tap
STS	Serological Test for Syphilis
STTEG	Stress Testing
THCEN	Thoracentesis
THCOSY	Thoracoscopy
TVS	Transvaginal Ultrasonography
TYMP	Tympanometry
UA	Urinalysis
ULT	Ultrasonography
VDA	Venous Digital Arteriography
WBC	White Blood Cell, White Blood Cell Count

3. ABBREVIATIONS FOR COMMON DIAGNOSTIC AND LABORATORY TESTS

Root	Meaning	Example
Abdomin/o	Abdomen	Abdominal
Actin/o	Light	Actinotherapy
Acou	Hear	Acoustic
Acu	Sharp, Abrupt	Acupressure
Aden/o	Gland	Adenosarcoma
Aero	Air	Aerobic
Alge/si	Pain	Analgesic
Amnio	Bowl	Amniocentesis
Andro	Masculine	Androgyny
Ankyl	Bent, Crooked	Ankylosis
Anter/o	Front	Anterointernal
Anthro	Man, Human	Philanthropic
Arteri/o	Artery	Arteriolsclerosis
Arthr/o	Joint	Arthritis
Asthm	Short of Breath	Asthmatic
Atri	Entry Chamber	Bariatrics
Audi/o	Hearing	Audiology
Auto	Self	Autoimmune
Bacteri	Bacteria	Antibacterial
Baro	Weight, Pressure	Baroreceptor
Bas/o, Basi/o	Base	Basophil
Bio	Life	Antibiotic
Brachi/o	Arm	Brachiocephalic
Bronch/i, bronch/o	Bronchus	Bronchial
Burs	Pocket	Bursitis
Carcin/o	Cancer	Carcinogen
Cardi/o	Heart	Cardiovascular
Carpo	Wrist	Carpometacarpal
Ceph/Cephal	Head	Cephaledema

Root	Meaning	Example
Cereb	Brain	Cerebellum
Chol/e	Bile	Choledochectomy
Col/o	Colon	Colonoscopy
Corp	Physical Body	Corpulent
Crin/o	Secretion	Endocrine
Cysto	Urinary, Bladder	Cystoplasty
Cyt/o	Cell	Cytogenetics
Dacty	Fingers, Digits	Dactylalgia
Dens/Dent	Tooth	Dentistry
Derm/a, Derm/o, Dermat/o	Skin	Dermatology
Digit	Finger, Toes	Orthodigita
Dors/i, Dors/o	Back or posterior	Dorsolumbar
Edem(a)	Excess	Podedema
Electro	Electricity	Electrocardiogram
Encephal/o	Brain	Electroencephalogram
Entero	Intestine	Enterobiasis
Etio	Cause	Etiology
Flect/Flex	Bend	Reflexogenic
Fract/Frag/Fring	Break	Fracture
Gastr/o	Stomach	Gastrointestinal
Gen	Origin	Genotoxic
Ger	Old	Gerontology
Gest	Bring Forth	Gestational
Gynec/o	Female	Gynecology
Hemat/o	Blood	Hematocystis
Hepat	Liver	Hepatitis
Hernia	Rupture	Herniation
Hist/o, histi/o	Tissue	Histoplasmosis
Hydro	Water	Hydrokinetic
Hypno	Sleep	Hypnotism

Root	Meaning	Example
Hyster/o	Uterus	Hysterectomy
Immun/o	Immune, Safe	Immunodeficiency
Intestin/o	Intestine	Renointestinal
Ject	Throw, Send	Injection
Junc/Jug/Jux	Join Together	Conjunctive
Lapar/o	Abdomen or Flank	Laparoscopy
Later/o	Side	Bilateral
Liga	Bind Together	Ligament
Lip/o	Fat	Liposuction
Lymph/o	Lymph Vessels	Lymphoma
Mal/i	Bad	Malignant
My/o	Muscle	Myocarditis
Narco	Numbness, Sleep	Narcolepsy
Neur/o	Nerve	Neurotransmitter
Ocul/o	Eye	Monocular
Ophthalm/o	Eyes	Ophthalmology
Optic/o, Opt/o	Seeing, Sight	Fiberoptics
Or/o	Mouth	Orolingual
Orth/o	Normal, Straight	Orthodontics
Ot/o	Ear	Epiotic
Path/o	Disease	Pathogen
Pharmac/o	Drug	Pharmacology
Psych	Mind	Psychiatric
Pulmon/o	Lungs	Pulmonary
Schiz/o	Split	Schizophrenia
Scolio	Bent, Crooked	Scoliosis
Sept/o	Infection	Antiseptic
Sono	Sound	Ultrasonography
Spir/o	Breathe	Respiration
Thorac/o	Chest/Thorax	Thoracic

Root	Meaning	Example
Thyr/o	Thyroid Gland	Hypothyroidism
Tox	Poison	Toxicology
Trachel/o	Neck	Trachelism
Trich/o	Hair	Trichopathy
Ventr/i, Ventr/o	Front of Body	Ventrolateral
Viscer/o, Viscera	Internal Organs	Visceroskeleton
Vivi	Life	Vivisection

4. COMMON MEDICAL PREFIXES

Prefix	Meaning	Example
A	Without	Atrophy
Ab	From	Abductor
Alg	Pain	Algesic
Ambi/Amphi	Both	Ambidextrous
An	Without	Anaerobic
Ana	Up, Again	Anabolism
Aniso	Unequal	Anisotropic
Ante	Before	Antepartum
Anti	Against	Antibodies
Apo	Upon	Aporepressor
Auto	Self	Autoimmune
Bi/Bin	Two	Binaural
Bio	Life	Biology
Brady	Slow	Bradypnea
Circum	Around	Circumcision
Con	Together	Conception
Contra	Opposed	Contraceptive
Cyte	Cell	Cytoglucopenia
De	Reverse	Defibrillate
Di	Two	Dicephalous
Dia	Thorough	Diapedesis
Diplo	Double	Diplomyelia
Dis	Undo	Dislocation
Dys	Difficult, Abnormal	Dyspnea
E/Ec/Ecto/Ek	Outside	Ectocornea
Em/En/Endo/Ent	Within	Endoskeleton
Epi	On	Epidural
Eso	Carry	Esophagus
Eu	Normal, Well	Euphoria

Prefix	Meaning	Example
Eury	Broad	Eurysomatic
Ex/Exo	Outside	Exophthalmos
Extra	Beyond	Extraphysiologic
Hapto	Bind	Haptoglobin
Hemi	Half	Hemiplegia
Hemo	Blood	Hemoglobin
Hept	Seven	Heptapeptide
Hetero	Different	Heterogenic
Homo	Same	Homogeneous
Hyper	Excessive	Hyperactivity
Hypo	Deficient	Hypoallergenic
Im/In	Into, Not	Intubate
Infra	Below, Under	Infrasonic
Inter	Among, Between	Intercerebral
Intra	Within	Intravenous
Intro	During	Introjection
Iso	Equal	Isoenzyme
Juxta	Adjacent	Juxtaintestinal
Macro/Magno/Mega	Large	Macroscopic
Mal	Bad	Malnutrition
Medi/Meso	Middle	Mesoderm
Mega/Megalo	Large	Megalocardia
Meta	After, Beyond	Metatarsus
Micro	Small	Microorganism
Multi	Many	Multinodular
Neo	New	Neonatal
Non	Not	Nontoxic
Nulli	None	Nulliparous
Ob	Before	Obstetrics
Onco	Tumor	Oncology

Prefix	Meaning	Example
Opt	Vision	Optometry
Pachy	Thick	Pachyblepharon
Pan	Total	Panarteritis
Para	Beside, Around	Parachordal
Pent	Five	Pentapeptide
Per	By, Through	Percutaneous
Peri	Surrounding	Perineurium
Pleo	More Than Usual	Pleonosteosis
Poly	Many	Polycystic
Post	After	Postoperative
Pre/Pro	Before	Preoperative
Pros/Prox	Beside	Proximolabial
Pseudo	FALSE	Pseudolipoma
Quar/Quad	Four	Quartisect
Re	Back	Reflux
Retro	Behind	Retroflexion
Semi	Half	Semimembranous
Sept	Seven	Septuplet
Sex	Six	Sextuplet
Sub	Under	Subcutaneous
Super/Supra	Above, Over	Suprascapular
Sym/Syn/Sys	Together, Joined	Symbiosis
Tachy	Rapid	Tachyarrhythmia
Tetra	Four	Tetraperomelia
Toxi	Poison	Toxicology
Trans	Across	Transfusion
Tri	Three	Tribasilar
Uni	One	Uniglandular
Ultra	Beyond	Ultrasonography

5. COMMON MEDICAL SUFFIXES

Suffix	Meaning	Example
Ache	Pain	Headache
Algia	Pain	Fibromyalgia
Ary	Pertaining to, Connected to	Coronary
Ase	Fermenter	Thioesterase
Cele	Hernia, Protrusion	Aerocele
Centesis	Surgical Puncture	Amniocentesis
Cidal	Killing	Suicidal
Coccus/Cocci	Spherical	Streptococci
Crit	To Separate	Plasmacrit
Cyte	Cell	Keratocyte
Desis	Fusion	Fasciodesis
Ectomy	Surgical Removal	Tonsillectomy
Emesis	Vomiting	Hyperemesis
Emia	Blood Condition	Leukemia
Esis	Condition	Paratenesis
Gen/Genic	Producing	Carcinogenic
Gram	Picture, Graph	Echocardiogram
Graph	Recording Instrument	Electrocardiograph
Graphy	Process of Recording	Tomography
Iasis	Full of	Psoriasis
Iatry	Physician, Treatment	Podiatry
Ician	One Who	Dietician
Ism	State of	Polymorphism
Itis	Inflammation	Laryngitis
Lepsy	Seizure	Epilepsy
Logist	Specialist	Anesthesiologist
Logy	Study of	Dermatology
Lysis	Dissolution	Urinalysis
Lytic	Destroy	Thrombolytic

Suffix	Meaning	Example
Malacia	Softening	Arteriomalacia
Megaly	Enlargement	Tracheomegaly
Meter	Measuring Instrument	Thermometer
Metry	Measuring	Spirometry
Morph	Shape	Ectomorph
Natal	Birth	Perinatal
Oid	Resembling	Fibroid
Oma	Tumor	Lymphoma
Opia	Vision	Myopia
Opsy	To View	Autopsy
Osis	Condition	Halitosis
Pathy	Disease	Osteopathy
Penia	Deficiency	Thrombocytopenia
Pepsia	Digestion	Dyspepsia
Pexy	Fixation	Orchidopexy
Phagia	Eating, Swallowing	Dysphagia
Phobia	Fear	Acrophobia
Plasia	Development	Achondroplasia
Plasm	Growth, Formation	Cytoplasm
Plasty	Surgical Repair	Rhinoplasty
Plegia	Paralysis	Paraplegia
Pnea	Breath	Apnea
Porosis	Passage	Osteoporosis
Ptosis	Prolapse	Gastroptosis
Ptysis	Spitting	Hemoptysis
Rrhagia	Excessive Discharge	Menometrorrhagia
Rrhea	Excessive Discharge	Gonorrhea
Scope	Exam Instrument	Endoscope
Scopy	Examining	Ophthalmoscopy
Spasm	Involuntary Contraction	Bronchospasm

Suffix	Meaning	Example
Stasis	Control, Stop	Hemostasis
Stomy	Surgical Opening	Colostomy
Therapy	Treatment	Chemotherapy
Tocia	Birth, Labor	Dystocia
Tome	Cutting Instrument	Myelotome
Tomy	Incision	Appendectomy
Trophy	Growth	Atrophy
Ule	Little	Nodule
Uria	Urine	Rubruria

Prescription Abbreviations

The following lists contain abbreviations related specifically to the administration of prescription medications.

Abbreviation	Meaning
)	without
1/2NS	half normal saline (0.45%)
a.c.	before meals
a.m.	morning
A.T.C.	around the clock
ad lib	freely
ad	up to
a.d.	right ear (*auris dextra*)
admov.	apply
Agit	shake, agitate
a.l.	left ear (*auris laeva*)
alt. h.	every other hour
Amp	ampule
Amt	amount
Aq	water
a.s.	left ear (*auris sininster*)
a.u.	both ears
B.S.	blood sugar
B.S.A.	body surface areas
b, bis	twice
b.d., b.i.d.	twice daily
B.M.	bowel movement
bol.	large dose
Bt	bedtime
BUCC	inside the cheek
Ç	with
cap., caps.	capsule
cc	with food
cc	cubic centimeter
cib.	food
D.W.	distilled water
D.A.W.	dispense as written

Abbreviation	Meaning
D/C, disc.	discontinue
dieb. alt.	every other day
dil.	dilute
disp.	dispense
div.	divide
e.m.p.	as directed
elix.	elixir
emuls.	emulsion
ex aq	in water
fl.	fluid
g	gram
gr	grain
gtt(s)	drops
H	hypodermic
h, hr	hour
h.s.	at bedtime
ID	in the skin
IM	into the muscle
inj.	injection
int.c.	between meals
IV	intravenously
IVPB	intravenous piggyback
L.A.S.	label as such
liq	liquor
lot.	lotion
M.	mix
m.,min.	a minimum
mane	in the morning
mcg	microgram
mEq	milliequivalent
mg	milligrams
mist.	mix (*mistura*)
mitte	send
mL	milliliter
nebul	spray
N.M.T.	not more than
noct.	at night
non rep.	only once, do not repeat

Abbreviation	Meaning
NS	normal saline (0.9%)
NTE	not to exceed
o	with
ø	without
o.p.d.	once per day
o_2	both eyes
O$_2$	oxygen
o.d.	right eye (*oculus dexter*)
o.s.	left eye (*oculus sinister*)
o.u.	both eyes (*oculus uterque*)
p.c.	after meals
pil	pill
p.m.	afternoon or evening
pig., pigm.	paint
p.o.	by mouth (orally)
p.r.	through the rectum
p r n	as needed (*pro re nata*)
q	every
q.a.d.	every other day
q.a.m.	every morning
q.d.	daily
q.d.s.	four times daily
q.h.s.	daily at bedtime
q.h., q.1h	every hour
q.2h, q.2°	every 2 hours
q.i.d.	four times a day
q.o.d.	every other day
q.p.m.	daily in the afternoon or evening
qqh	every four hours
q.s.	a sufficient quantity
R	rectal
rep.	repeats
s.a.	according to your judgment
SC, subc	under the skin
sig.	label it as/write directions
SL	under the tongue
ss	one half
stat	immediately

Abbreviation	Meaning
supp	suppository
susp	suspension
syr	syrup
T	temperature
t.i.w.	three times weekly
tabs	tablets
tal., t	such
tbsp	tablespoon (15ml)
t.d.s.	three times daily
t.i.d.	three times daily
top.	topically
tinc.	tincture
tsp	teaspoon (5ml)
u.d.	as directed (*ut dictum*)
ung.	ointment
vag.	vaginally
w/	with
w/o	without
wf	with food (meals)
X	times
#	number
†	one
††	two
†††	three

Anatomy Images

SKELETAL SYSTEM

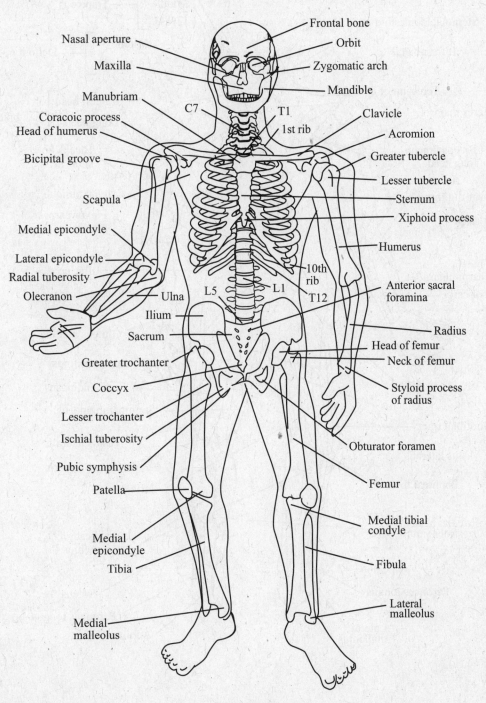

Nasal aperture
Maxilla
Manubriam
Coracoic process
Head of humerus
Bicipital groove
Scapula
Medial epicondyle
Lateral epicondyle
Radial tuberosity
Olecranon
Ulna
Ilium
Sacrum
Greater trochanter
Coccyx
Lesser trochanter
Ischial tuberosity
Pubic symphysis
Patella
Medial epicondyle
Tibia
Medial malleolus

C7
T1
1st rib
L5
L1
T12
10th rib

Frontal bone
Orbit
Zygomatic arch
Mandible
Clavicle
Acromion
Greater tubercle
Lesser tubercle
Sternum
Xiphoid process
Humerus
Anterior sacral foramina
Radius
Head of femur
Neck of femur
Styloid process of radius
Obturator foramen
Femur
Medial tibial condyle
Fibula
Lateral malleolus

SUPERFICIAL MUSCLE SYSTEM

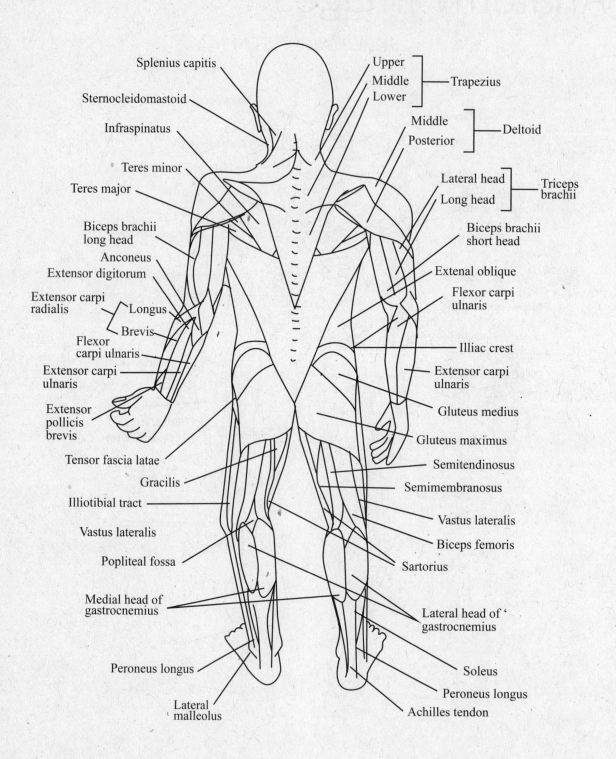

Splenius capitis

Sternocleidomastoid

Infraspinatus

Teres minor

Teres major

Biceps brachii
long head

Anconeus

Extensor digitorum

Extensor carpi
radialis

Longus

Brevis

Flexor
carpi ulnaris

Extensor carpi
ulnaris

Extensor
pollicis
brevis

Tensor fascia latae

Gracilis

Illiotibial tract

Vastus lateralis

Popliteal fossa

Medial head of
gastrocnemius

Peroneus longus

Lateral
malleolus

Upper
Middle
Lower

Trapezius

Middle
Posterior

Deltoid

Lateral head
Long head

Triceps
brachii

Biceps brachii
short head

Extenal oblique

Flexor carpi
ulnaris

Illiac crest

Extensor carpi
ulnaris

Gluteus medius

Gluteus maximus

Semitendinosus

Semimembranosus

Vastus lateralis

Biceps femoris

Sartorius

Lateral head of
gastrocnemius

Soleus

Peroneus longus

Achilles tendon

TYPE OF MUSCLE

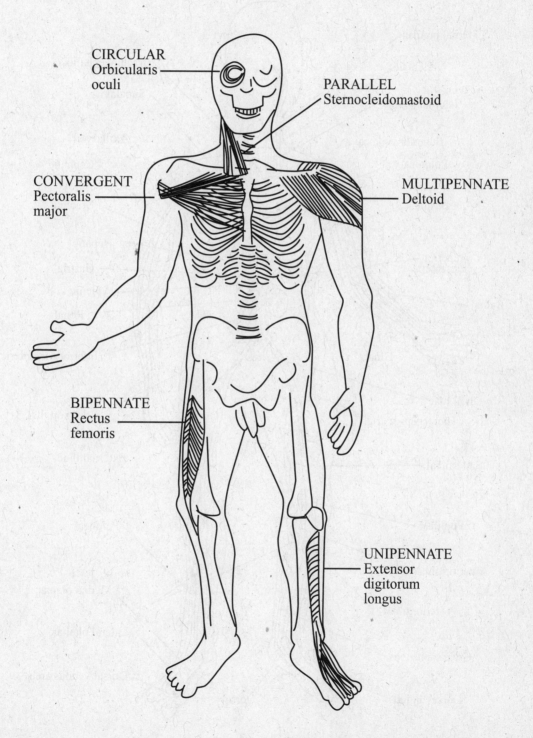

CIRCULAR
Orbicularis
oculi

PARALLEL
Sternocleidomastoid

CONVERGENT
Pectoralis
major

MULTIPENNATE
Deltoid

BIPENNATE
Rectus
femoris

UNIPENNATE
Extensor
digitorum
longus

CARDIOVASCULAR SYSTEM
VEINS

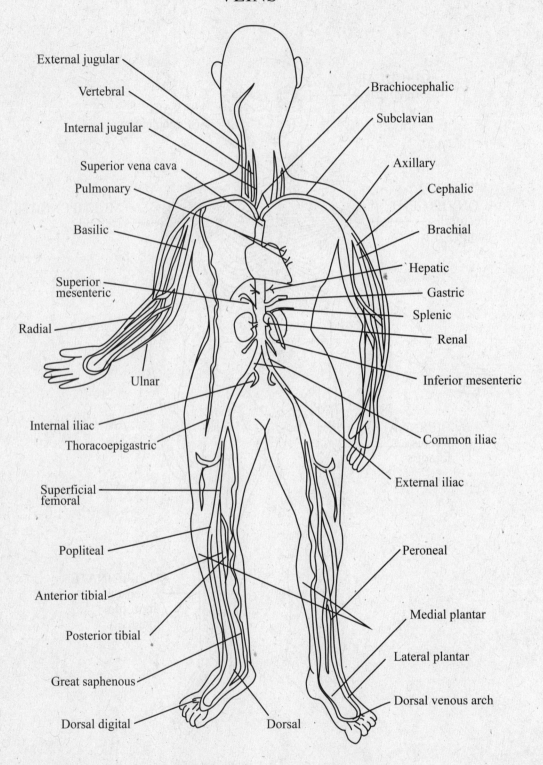

External jugular

Vertebral

Internal jugular

Superior vena cava

Pulmonary

Basilic

Superior mesenteric

Radial

Ulnar

Internal iliac

Thoracoepigastric

Superficial femoral

Popliteal

Anterior tibial

Posterior tibial

Great saphenous

Dorsal digital

Dorsal

Brachiocephalic

Subclavian

Axillary

Cephalic

Brachial

Hepatic

Gastric

Splenic

Renal

Inferior mesenteric

Common iliac

External iliac

Peroneal

Medial plantar

Lateral plantar

Dorsal venous arch

CARDIOVASCULAR SYSTEM
ARTERIES

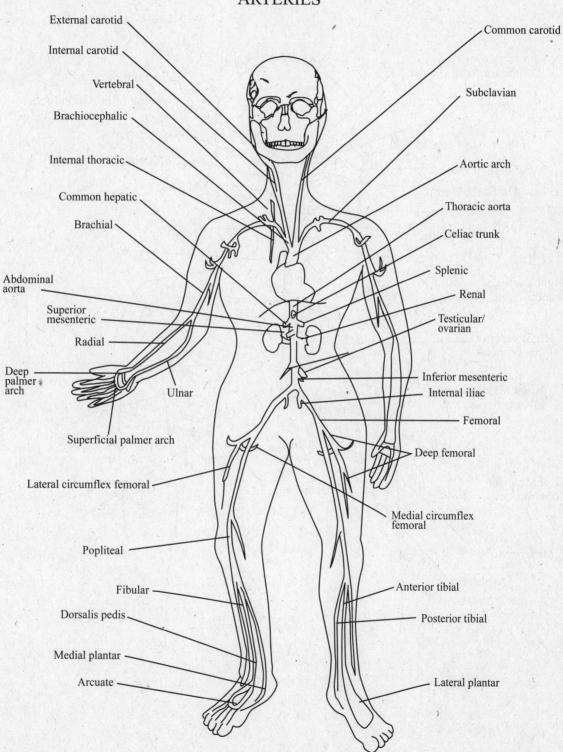

External carotid

Internal carotid

Vertebral

Brachiocephalic

Internal thoracic

Common hepatic

Brachial

Abdominal aorta

Superior mesenteric

Radial

Deep palmer arch

Ulnar

Superficial palmer arch

Lateral circumflex femoral

Popliteal

Fibular

Dorsalis pedis

Medial plantar

Arcuate

Common carotid

Subclavian

Aortic arch

Thoracic aorta

Celiac trunk

Splenic

Renal

Testicular/ovarian

Inferior mesenteric

Internal iliac

Femoral

Deep femoral

Medial circumflex femoral

Anterior tibial

Posterior tibial

Lateral plantar

RESPIRATORY SYSTEM

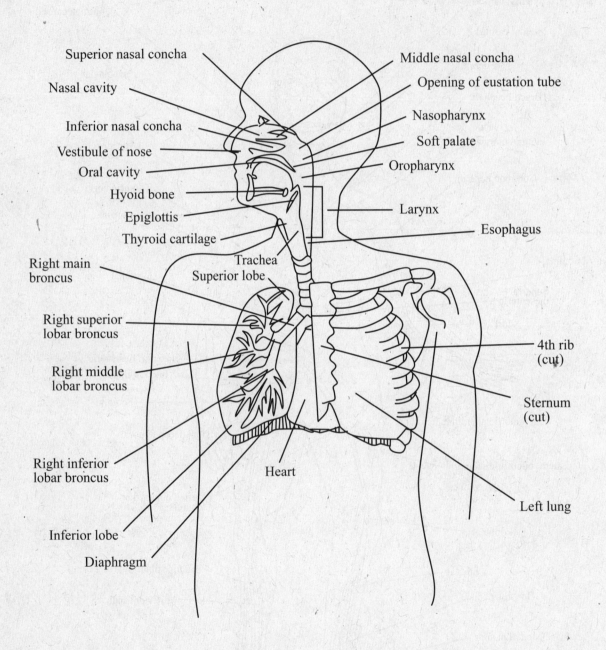

Superior nasal concha

Nasal cavity

Inferior nasal concha

Vestibule of nose

Oral cavity

Hyoid bone

Epiglottis

Thyroid cartilage

Right main broncus

Right superior lobar broncus

Right middle lobar broncus

Right inferior lobar broncus

Inferior lobe

Diaphragm

Middle nasal concha

Opening of eustation tube

Nasopharynx

Soft palate

Oropharynx

Larynx

Esophagus

Trachea

Superior lobe

4th rib (cut)

Sternum (cut)

Left lung

Heart

LYMPHATIC SYSTEM

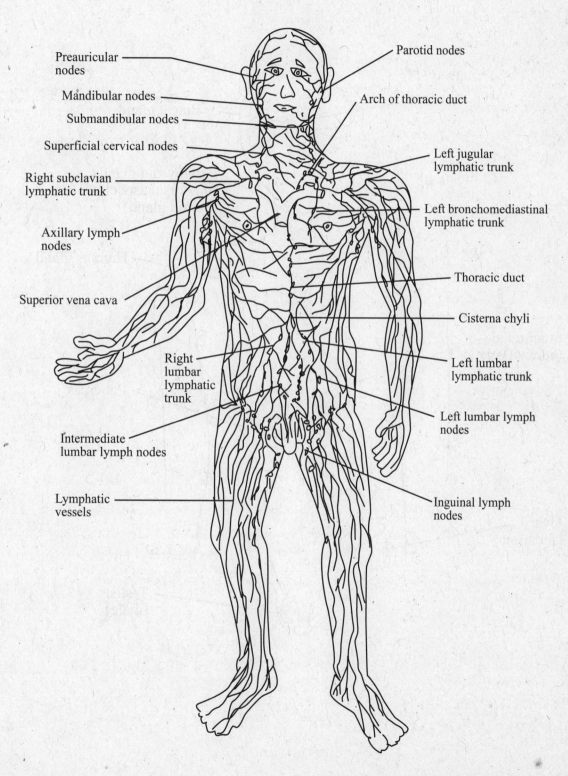

Preauricular nodes

Mandibular nodes

Submandibular nodes

Superficial cervical nodes

Right subclavian lymphatic trunk

Axillary lymph nodes

Superior vena cava

Right lumbar lymphatic trunk

Intermediate lumbar lymph nodes

Lymphatic vessels

Parotid nodes

Arch of thoracic duct

Left jugular lymphatic trunk

Left bronchomediastinal lymphatic trunk

Thoracic duct

Cisterna chyli

Left lumbar lymphatic trunk

Left lumbar lymph nodes

Inguinal lymph nodes

ENDOCRINE SYSTEM

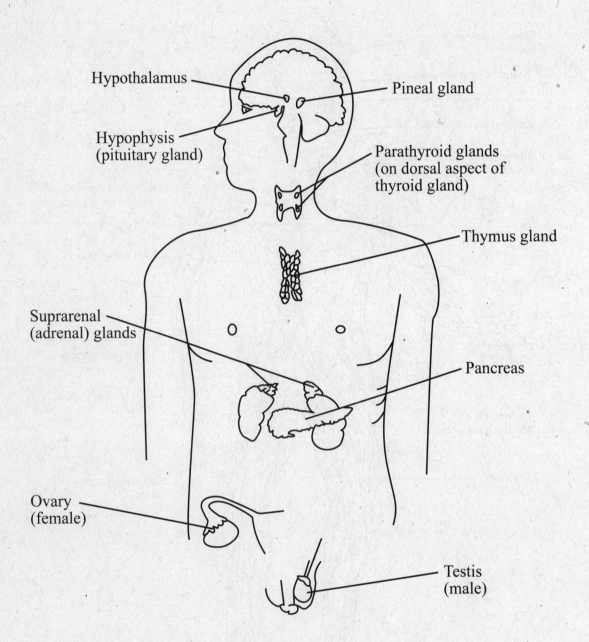

Hypothalamus

Pineal gland

Hypophysis
(pituitary gland)

Parathyroid glands
(on dorsal aspect of
thyroid gland)

Thymus gland

Suprarenal
(adrenal) glands

Pancreas

Ovary
(female)

Testis
(male)

DIGESTIVE SYSTEM

Gastrointestinal

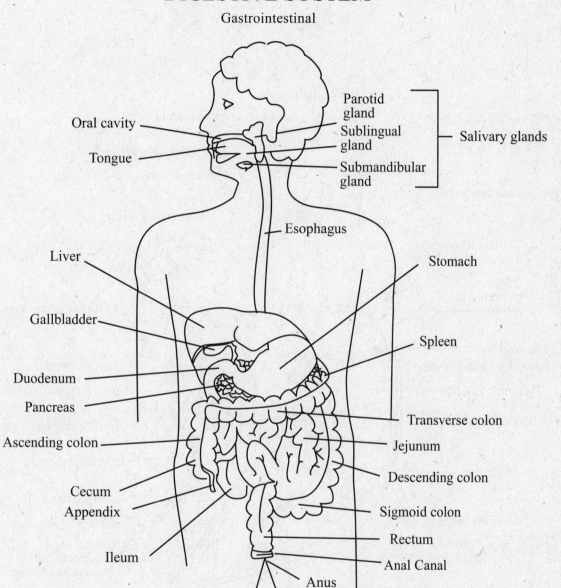

Oral cavity

Tongue

Parotid gland

Sublingual gland

Submandibular gland

Salivary glands

Esophagus

Liver

Stomach

Gallbladder

Spleen

Duodenum

Pancreas

Transverse colon

Ascending colon

Jejunum

Descending colon

Cecum

Appendix

Sigmoid colon

Rectum

Ileum

Anal Canal

Anus

THE HEART

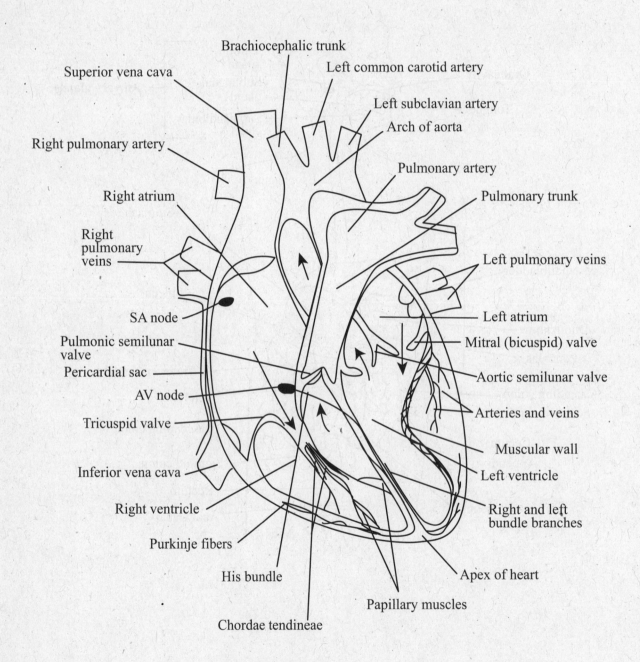

Brachiocephalic trunk

Left common carotid artery

Superior vena cava

Left subclavian artery

Arch of aorta

Right pulmonary artery

Pulmonary artery

Right atrium

Pulmonary trunk

Right pulmonary veins

Left pulmonary veins

SA node

Left atrium

Pulmonic semilunar valve

Mitral (bicuspid) valve

Pericardial sac

Aortic semilunar valve

AV node

Arteries and veins

Tricuspid valve

Muscular wall

Inferior vena cava

Left ventricle

Right ventricle

Right and left bundle branches

Purkinje fibers

Apex of heart

His bundle

Papillary muscles

Chordae tendineae

SPINE

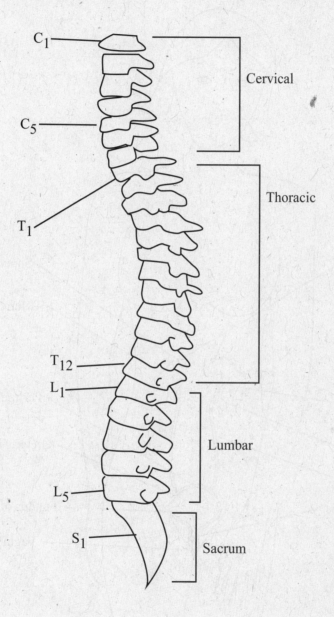

C₁

C₅

T₁

Cervical

Thoracic

T₁₂

L₁

Lumbar

L₅

S₁

Sacrum

URINARY TRACT

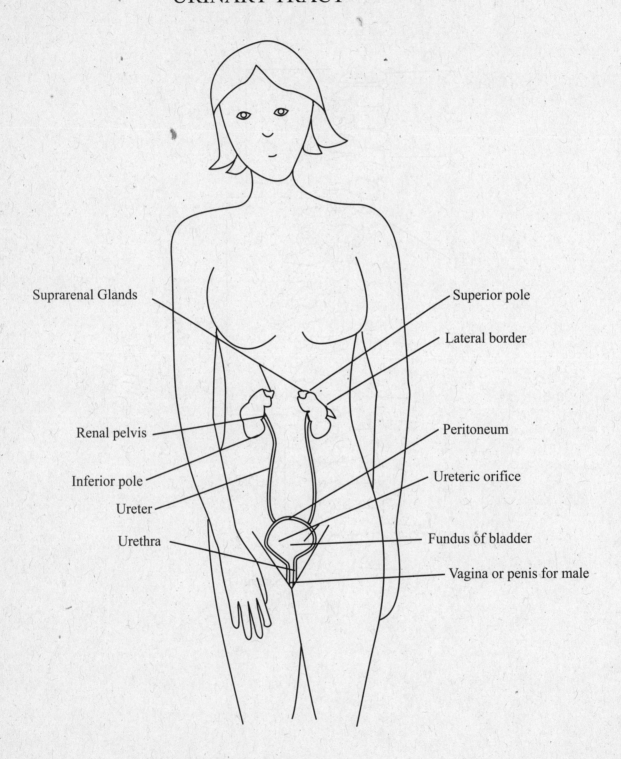

Suprarenal Glands

Superior pole

Lateral border

Renal pelvis

Peritoneum

Inferior pole

Ureteric orifice

Ureter

Urethra

Fundus of bladder

Vagina or penis for male

DERMATOMES

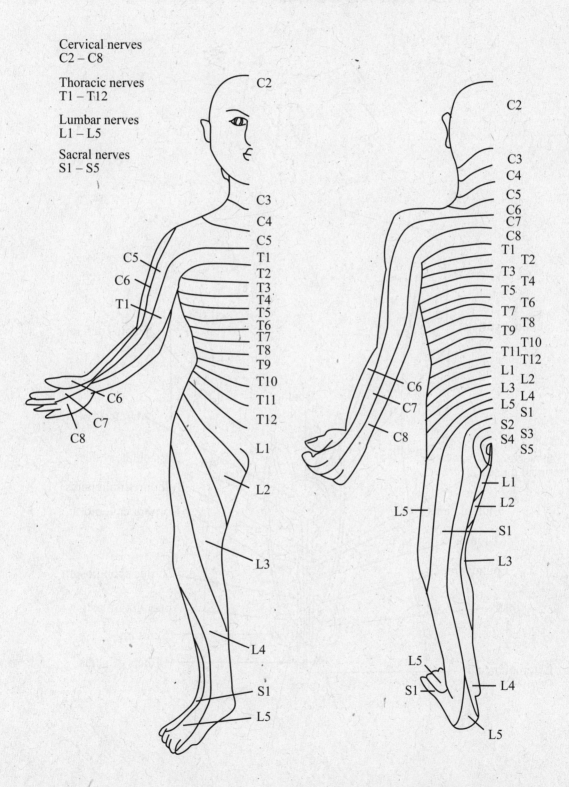

Cervical nerves
C2 – C8

Thoracic nerves
T1 – T12

Lumbar nerves
L1 – L5

Sacral nerves
S1 – S5

MALE REPRODUCTIVE SYSTEM

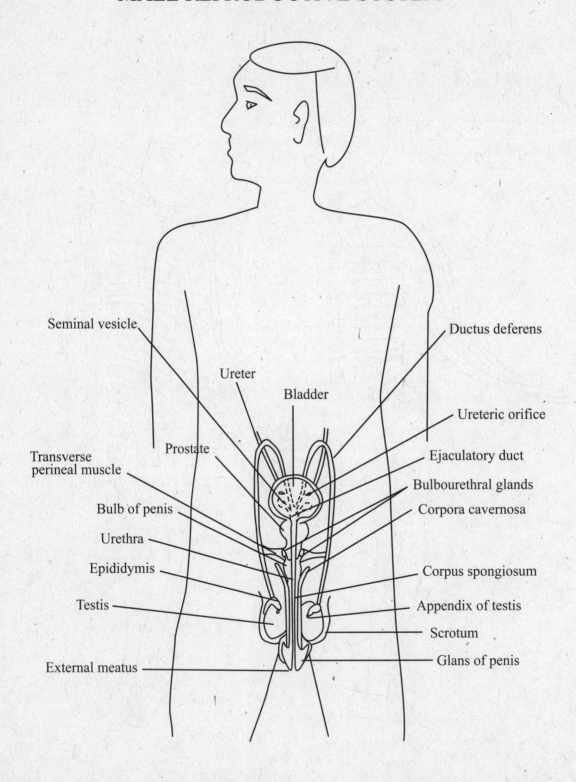

Seminal vesicle

Ureter

Bladder

Ductus deferens

Ureteric orifice

Ejaculatory duct

Prostate

Bulbourethral glands

Transverse
perineal muscle

Corpora cavernosa

Bulb of penis

Urethra

Epididymis

Corpus spongiosum

Testis

Appendix of testis

Scrotum

External meatus

Glans of penis

FEMALE REPRODUCTIVE SYSTEM

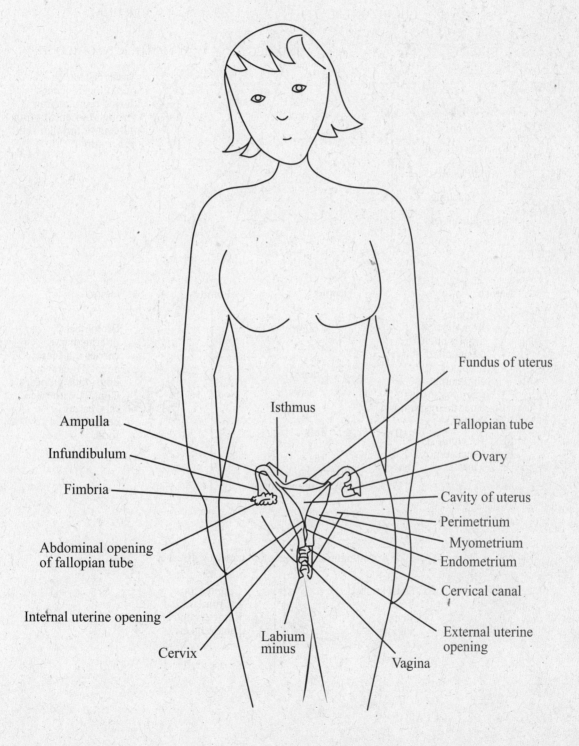

Fundus of uterus

Isthmus

Ampulla

Fallopian tube

Infundibulum

Ovary

Fimbria

Cavity of uterus

Perimetrium

Myometrium

Endometrium

Abdominal opening
of fallopian tube

Cervical canal

Internal uterine opening

External uterine
opening

Cervix

Labium
minus

Vagina

MODES OF DISEASE TRANSMISSION

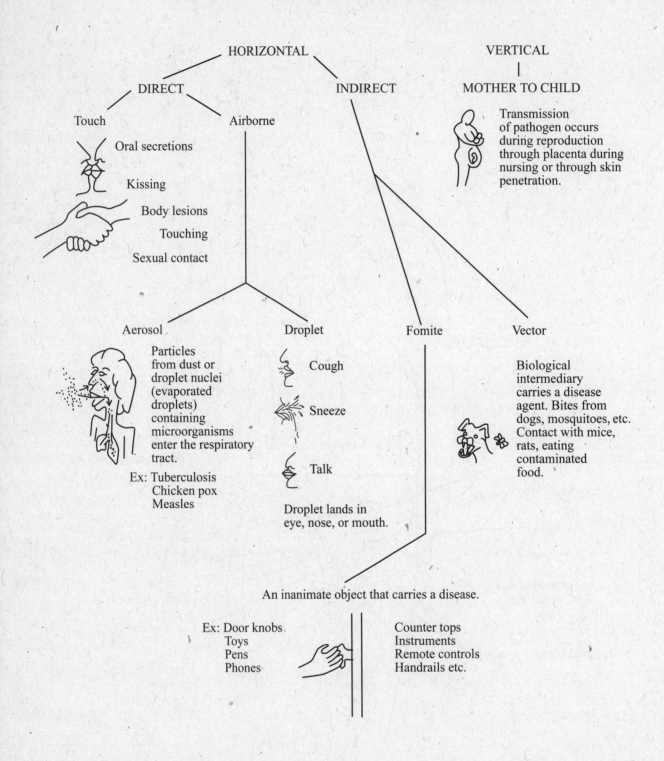

HORIZONTAL

VERTICAL

DIRECT INDIRECT MOTHER TO CHILD

Touch Airborne

Oral secretions

Kissing

Body lesions

Touching

Sexual contact

Transmission of pathogen occurs during reproduction through placenta during nursing or through skin penetration.

Aerosol Droplet Fomite Vector

Particles from dust or droplet nuclei (evaporated droplets) containing microorganisms enter the respiratory tract.

Ex: Tuberculosis
Chicken pox
Measles

Cough

Sneeze

Talk

Droplet lands in eye, nose, or mouth.

Biological intermediary carries a disease agent. Bites from dogs, mosquitoes, etc. Contact with mice, rats, eating contaminated food.

An inanimate object that carries a disease.

Ex: Door knobs
Toys
Pens
Phones

Counter tops
Instruments
Remote controls
Handrails etc.

CROSS SECTION OF SKIN

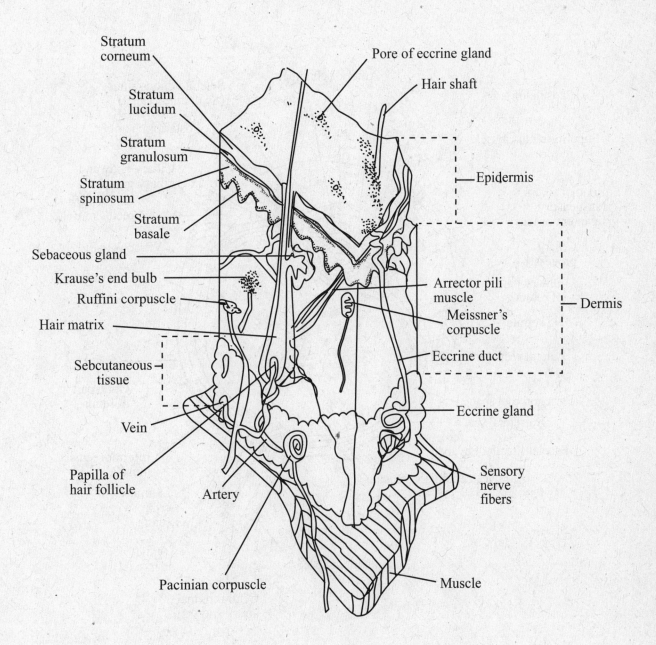

Stratum corneum

Stratum lucidum

Stratum granulosum

Stratum spinosum

Stratum basale

Sebaceous gland

Krause's end bulb

Ruffini corpuscle

Hair matrix

Sebcutaneous tissue

Vein

Papilla of hair follicle

Artery

Pacinian corpuscle

Pore of eccrine gland

Hair shaft

Epidermis

Arrector pili muscle

Meissner's corpuscle

Eccrine duct

Dermis

Eccrine gland

Sensory nerve fibers

Muscle

THE EYEBALL

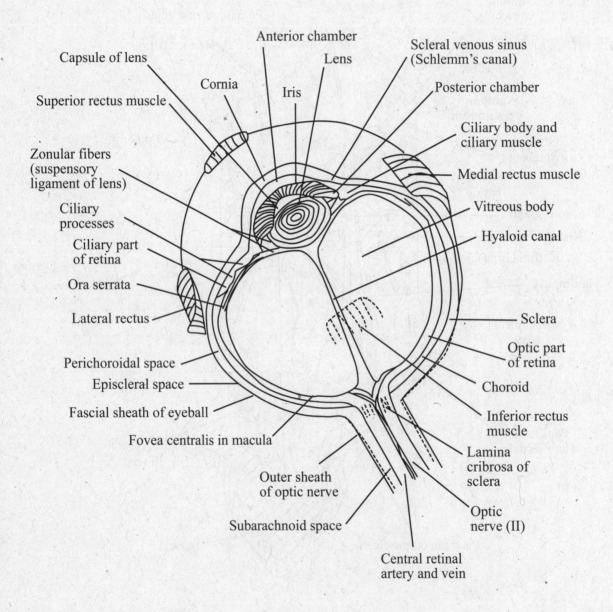

Anterior chamber

Capsule of lens

Scleral venous sinus
(Schlemm's canal)

Lens

Cornia

Posterior chamber

Superior rectus muscle

Iris

Ciliary body and
ciliary muscle

Zonular fibers
(suspensory
ligament of lens)

Medial rectus muscle

Vitreous body

Ciliary
processes

Hyaloid canal

Ciliary part
of retina

Ora serrata

Sclera

Lateral rectus

Optic part
of retina

Perichoroidal space

Choroid

Episcleral space

Inferior rectus
muscle

Fascial sheath of eyeball

Fovea centralis in macula

Lamina
cribrosa of
sclera

Outer sheath
of optic nerve

Optic
nerve (II)

Subarachnoid space

Central retinal
artery and vein

ANATOMY OF THE EAR

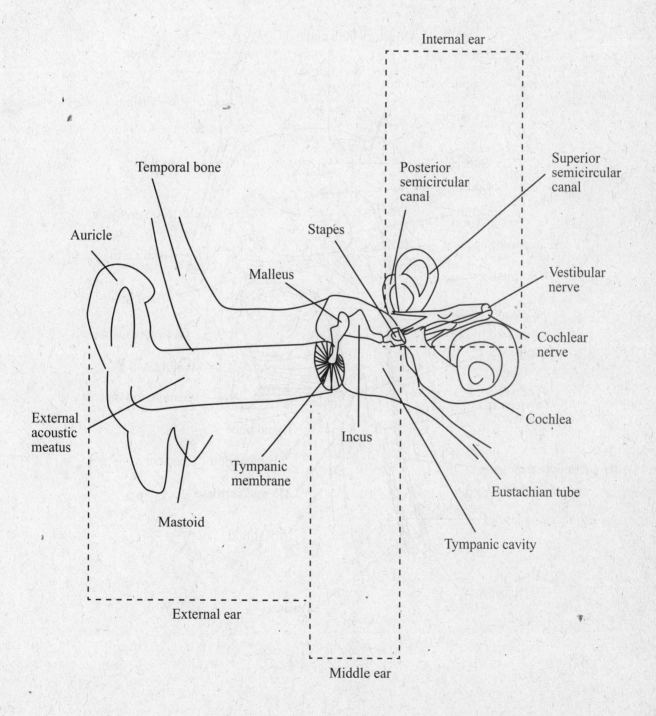

Internal ear

Temporal bone

Posterior semicircular canal

Superior semicircular canal

Stapes

Auricle

Malleus

Vestibular nerve

Cochlear nerve

External acoustic meatus

Incus

Cochlea

Tympanic membrane

Eustachian tube

Mastoid

Tympanic cavity

External ear

Middle ear

NASAL CAVITY

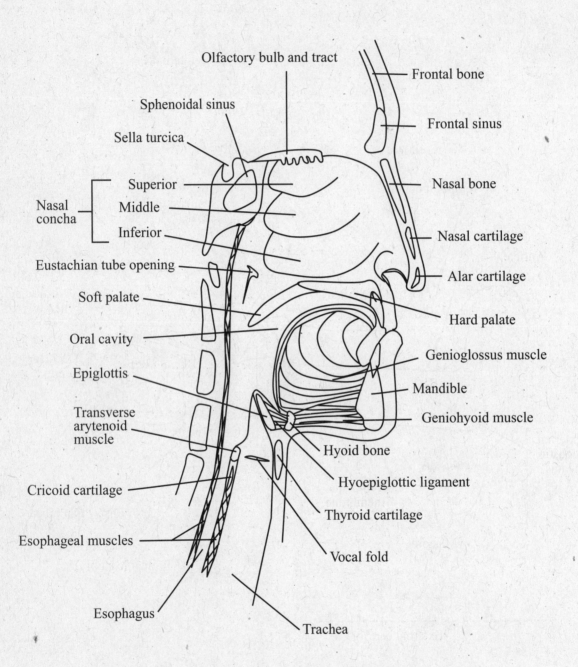

Olfactory bulb and tract

Sphenoidal sinus

Sella turcica

Superior

Nasal concha { Middle

Inferior

Eustachian tube opening

Soft palate

Oral cavity

Epiglottis

Transverse arytenoid muscle

Cricoid cartilage

Esophageal muscles

Esophagus

Frontal bone

Frontal sinus

Nasal bone

Nasal cartilage

Alar cartilage

Hard palate

Genioglossus muscle

Mandible

Geniohyoid muscle

Hyoid bone

Hyoepiglottic ligament

Thyroid cartilage

Vocal fold

Trachea

SCALE OF PAIN INTENSITY

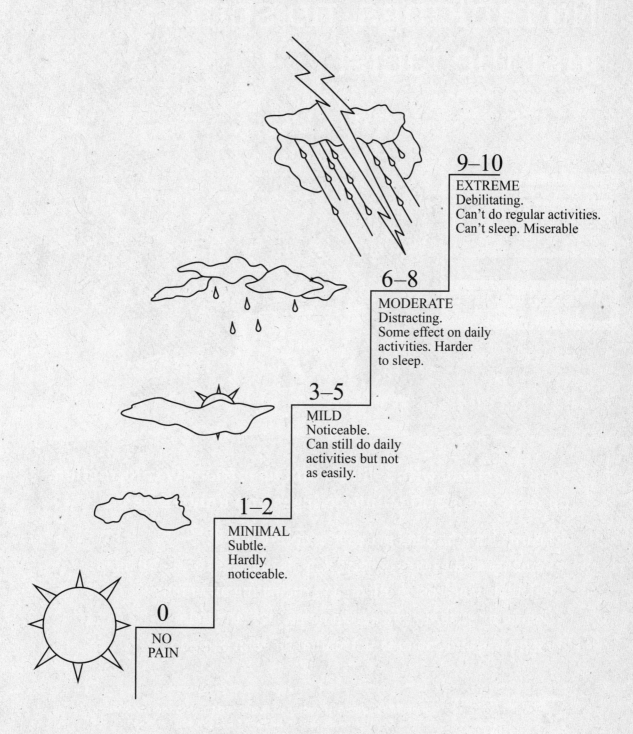

9–10
EXTREME
Debilitating.
Can't do regular activities.
Can't sleep. Miserable

6–8
MODERATE
Distracting.
Some effect on daily
activities. Harder
to sleep.

3–5
MILD
Noticeable.
Can still do daily
activities but not
as easily.

1–2
MINIMAL
Subtle.
Hardly
noticeable.

0
**NO
PAIN**

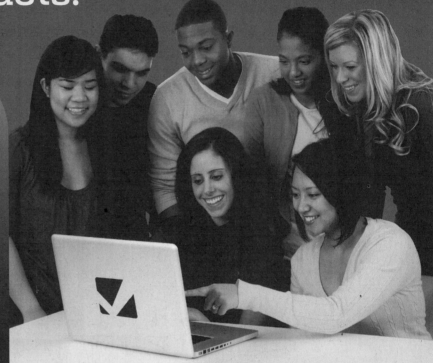
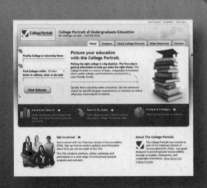
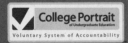